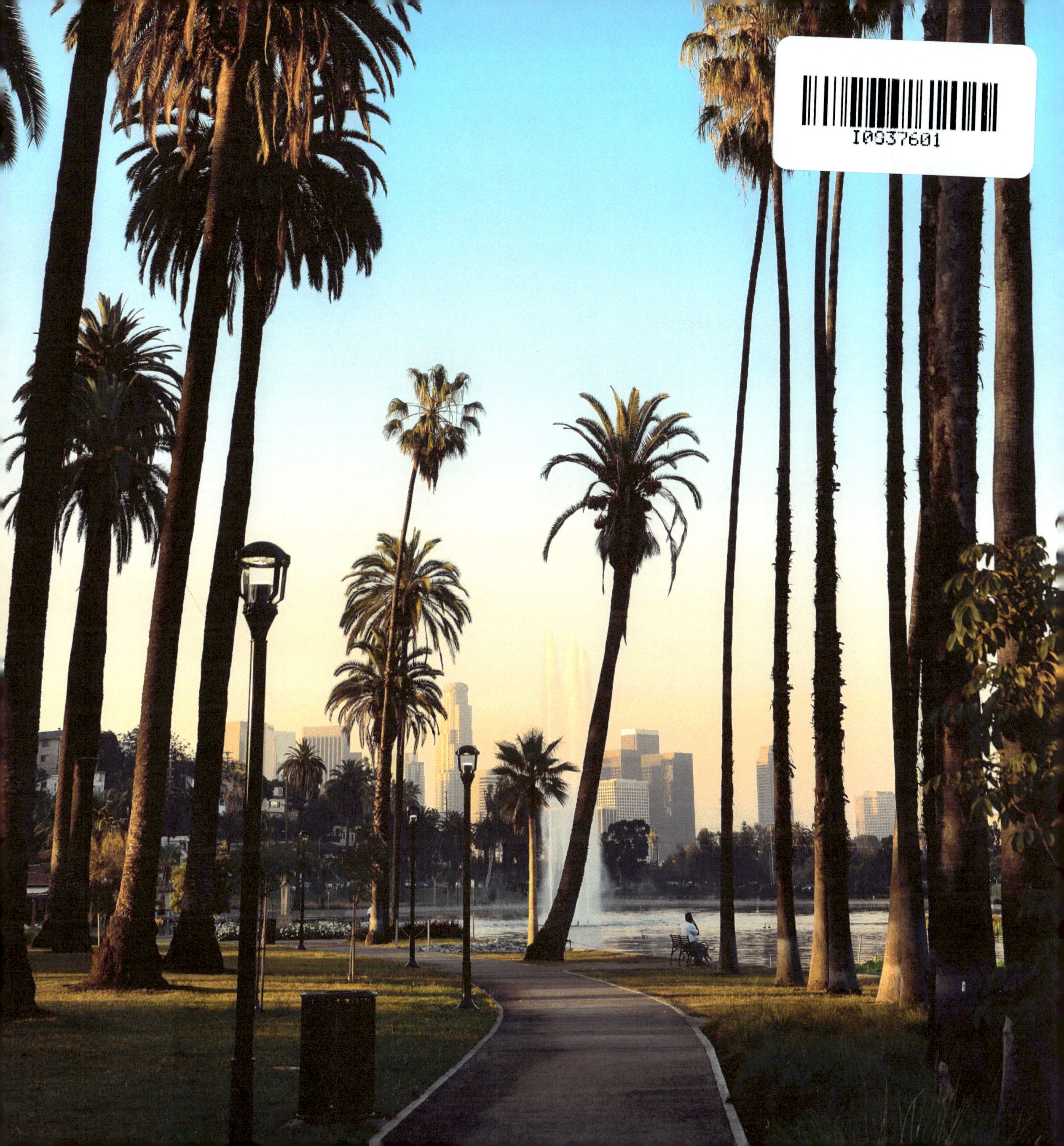

I0037601

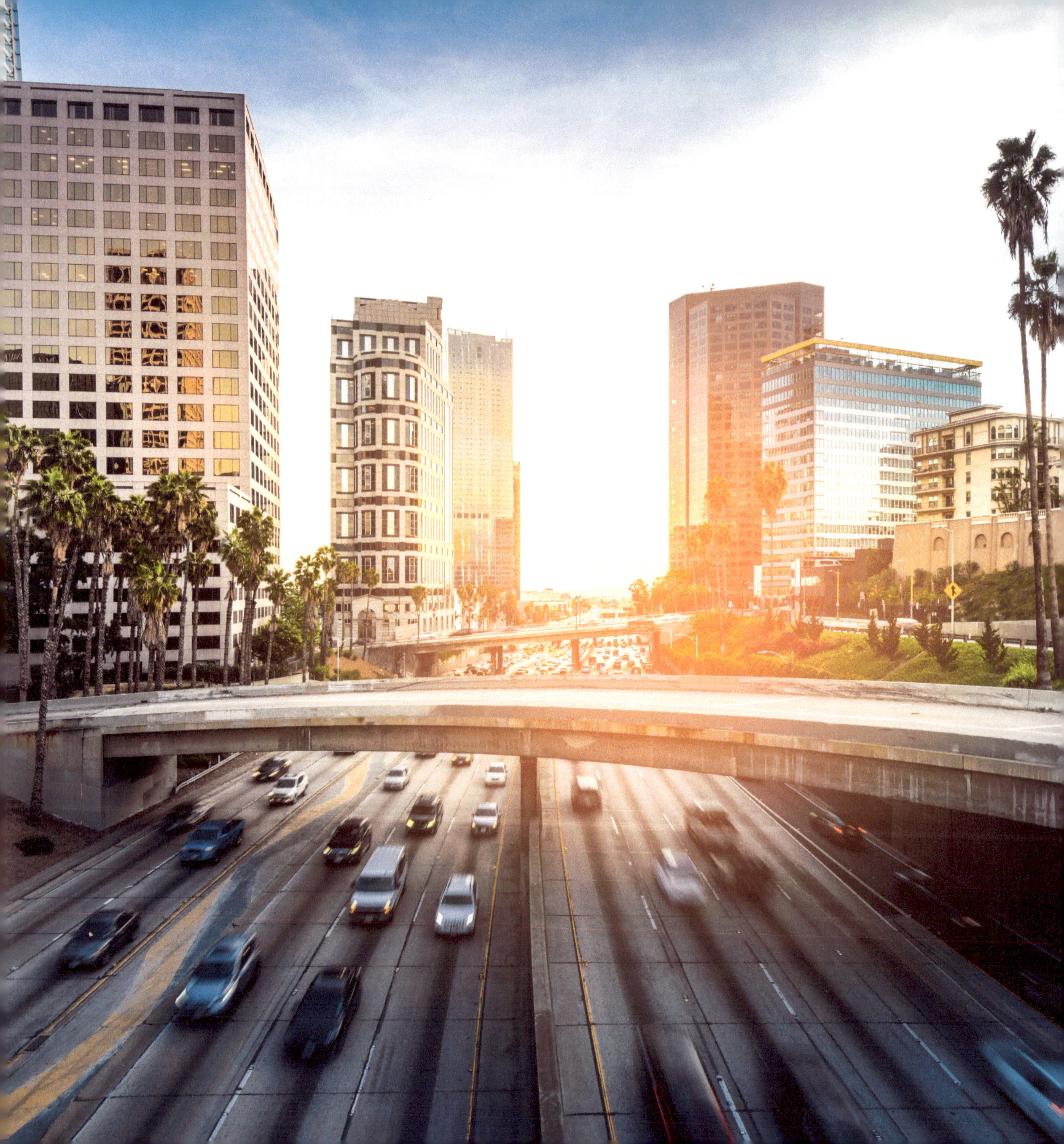

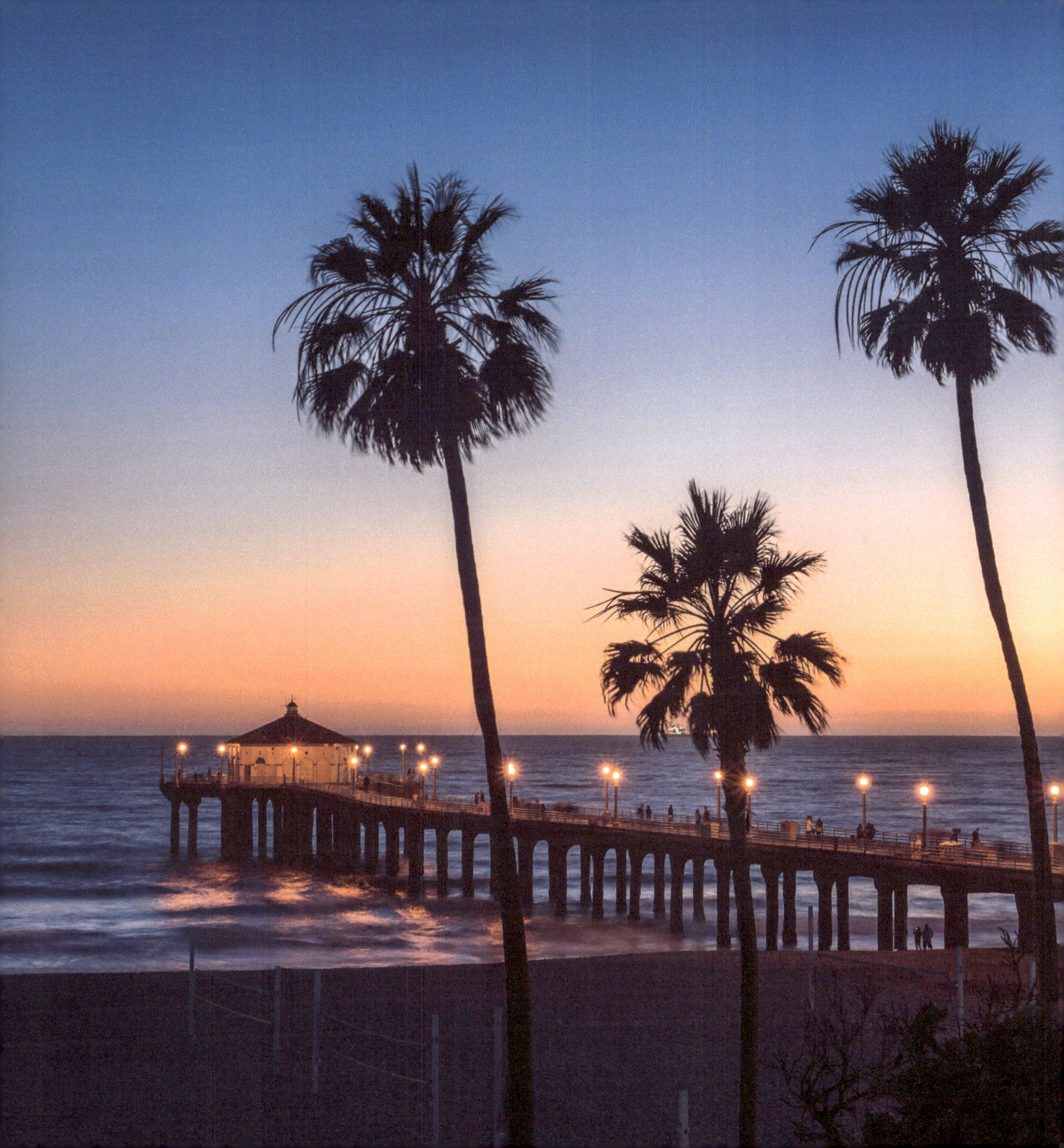

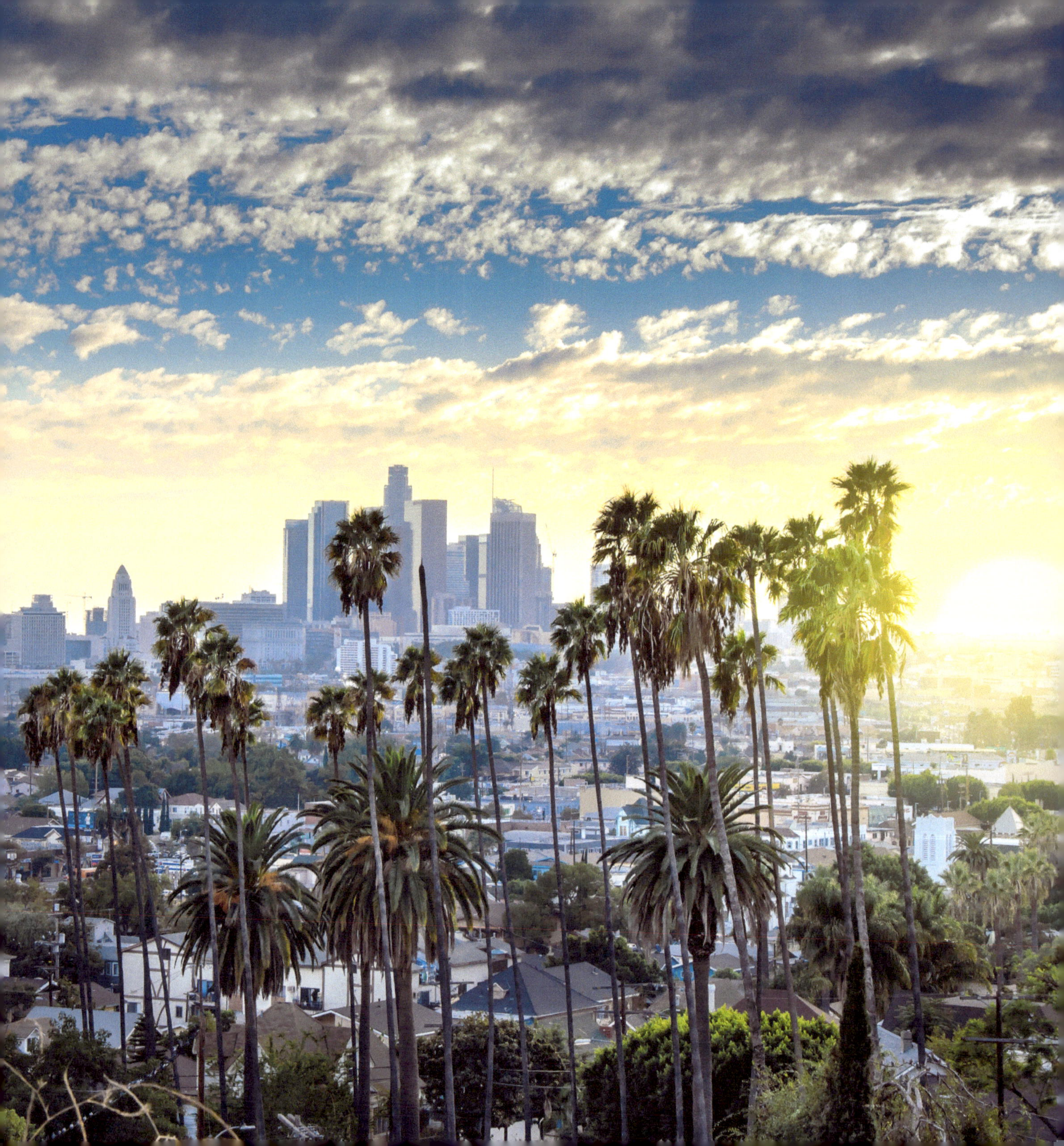

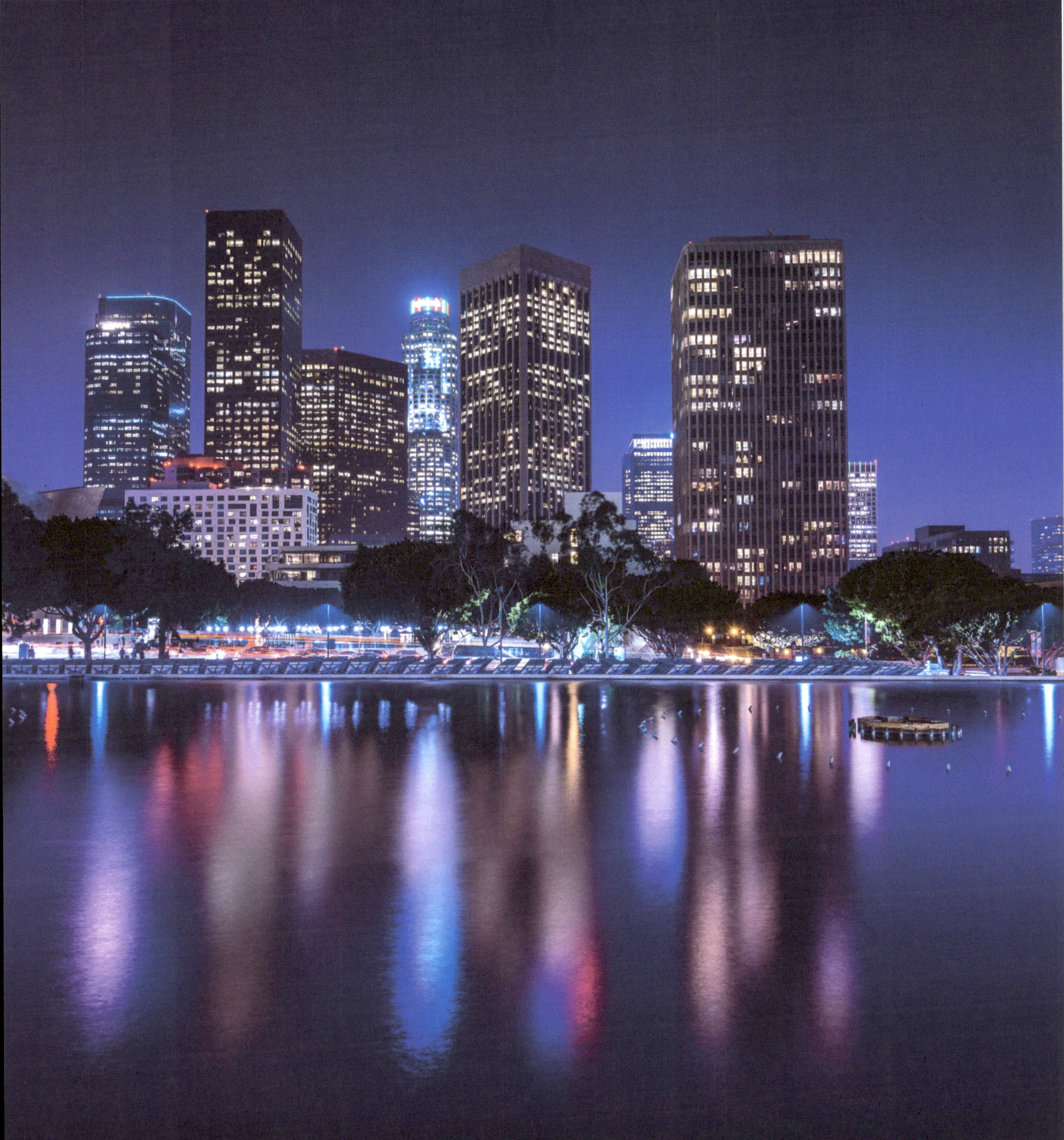

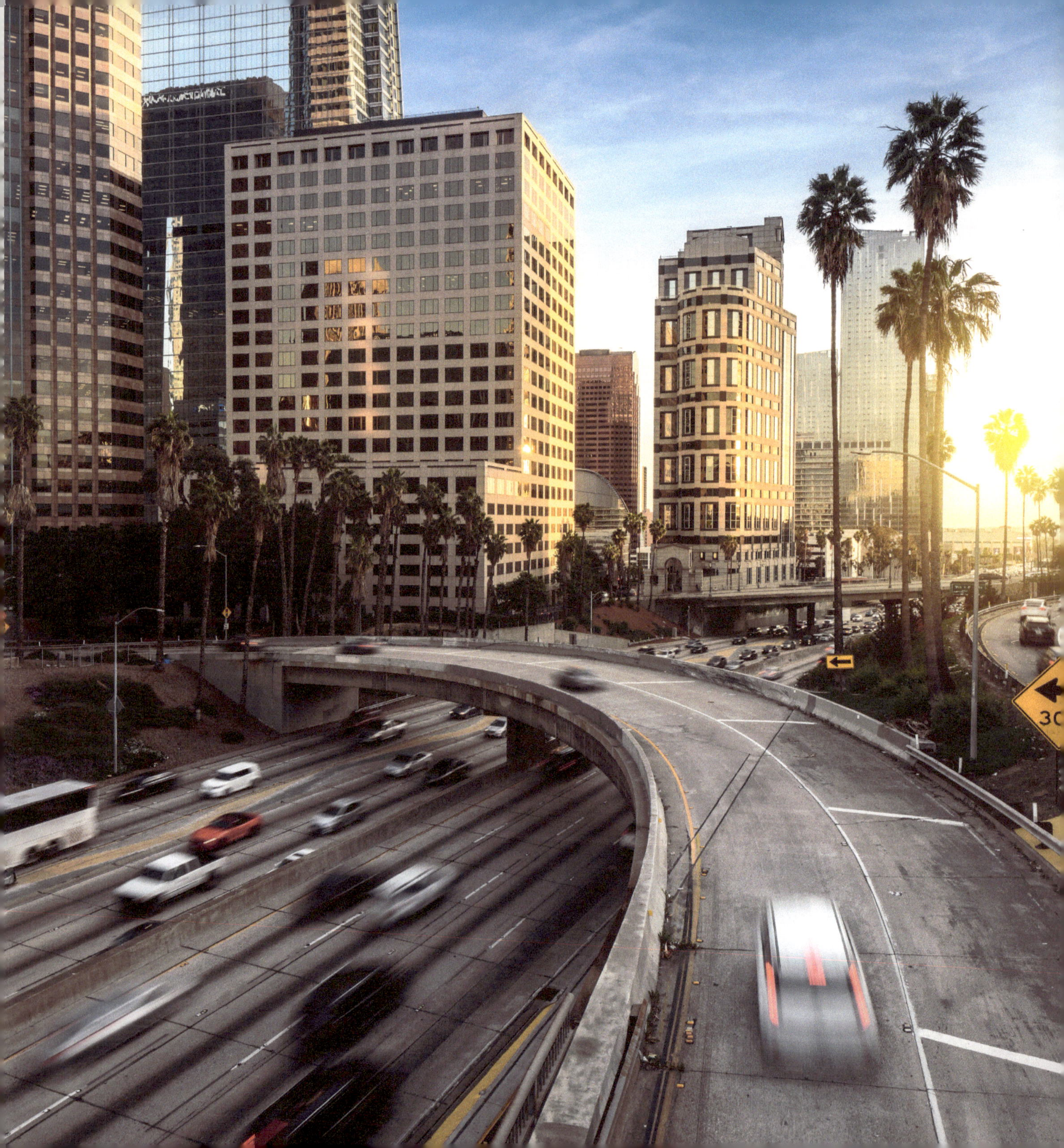

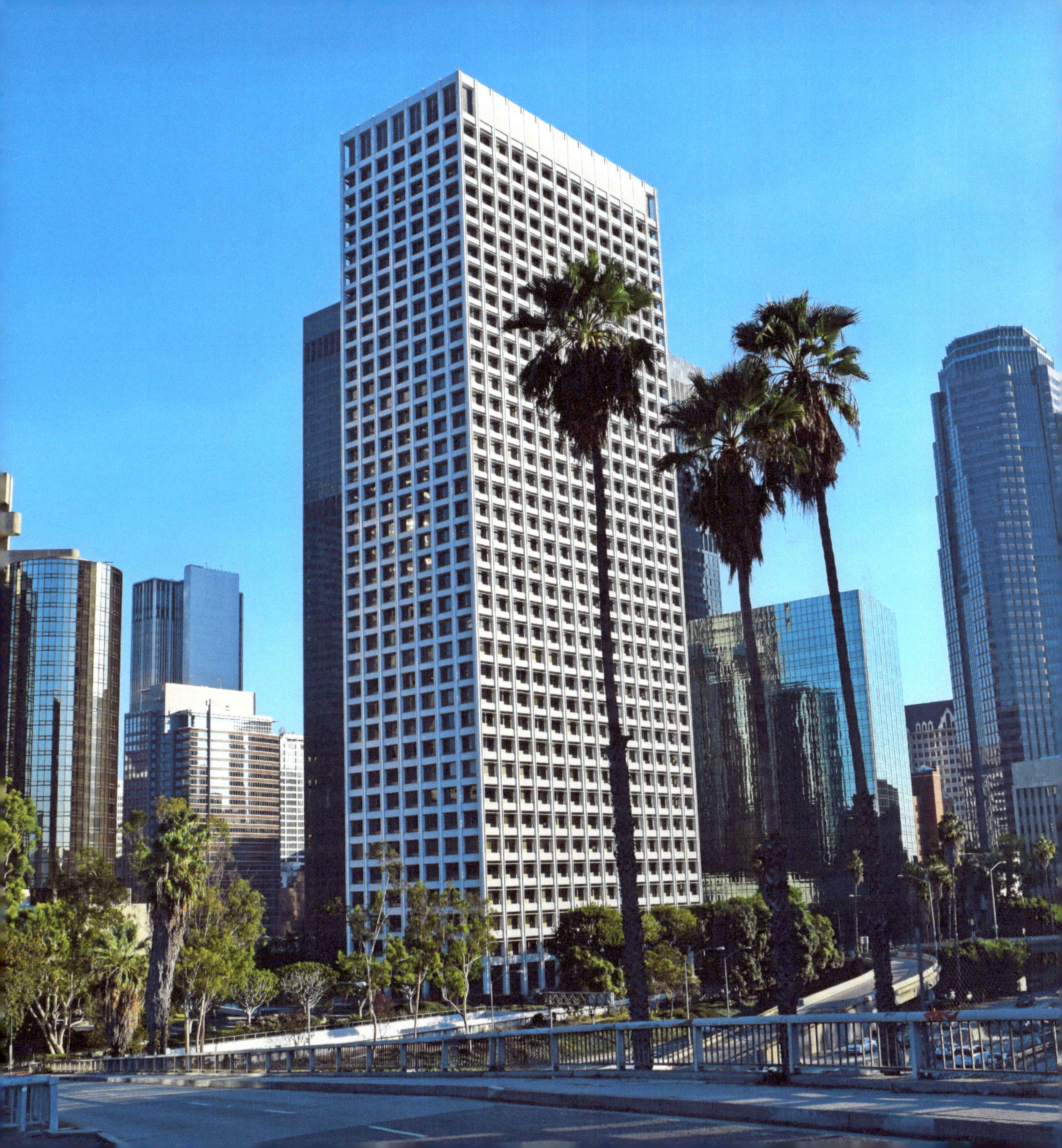

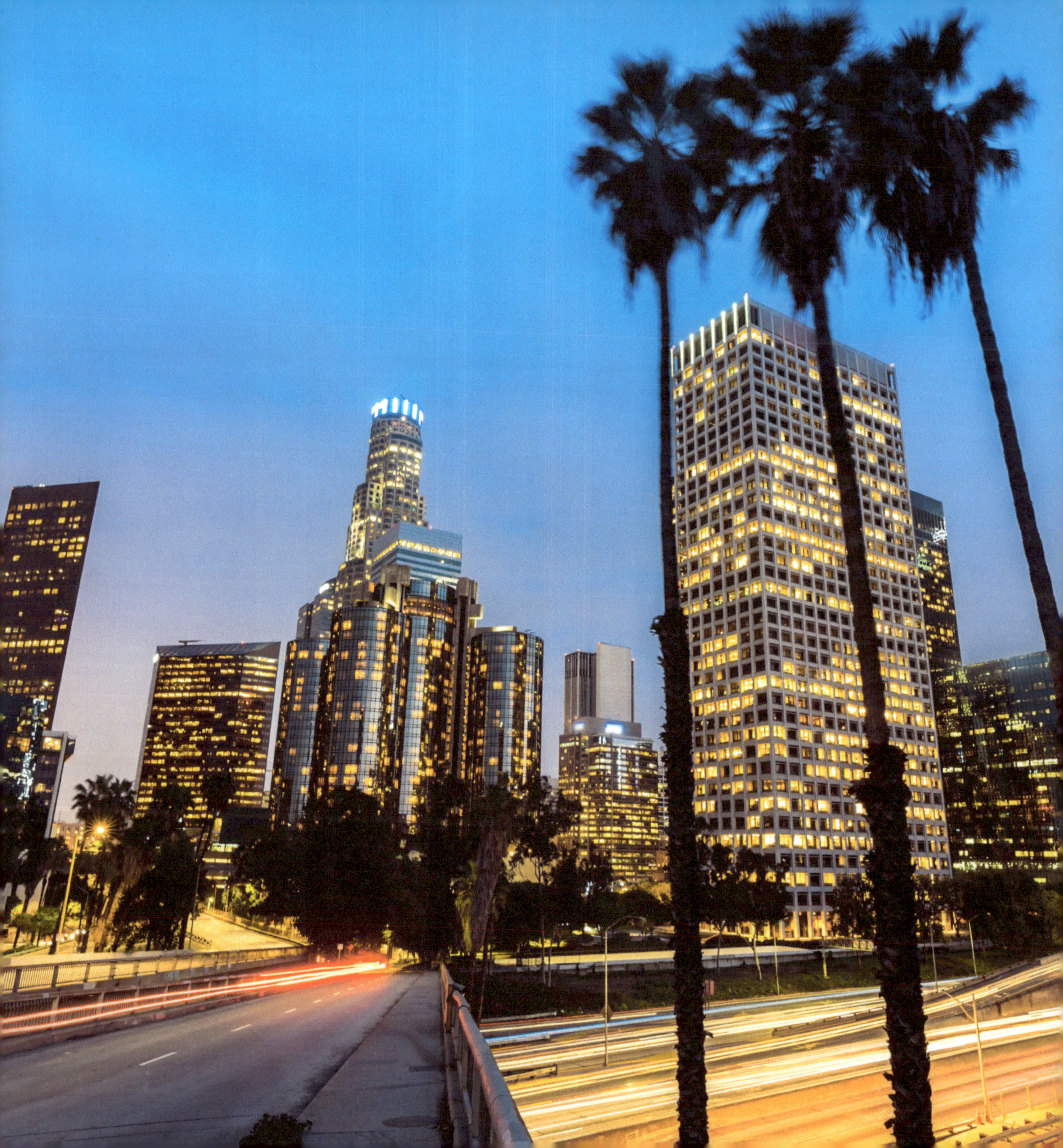

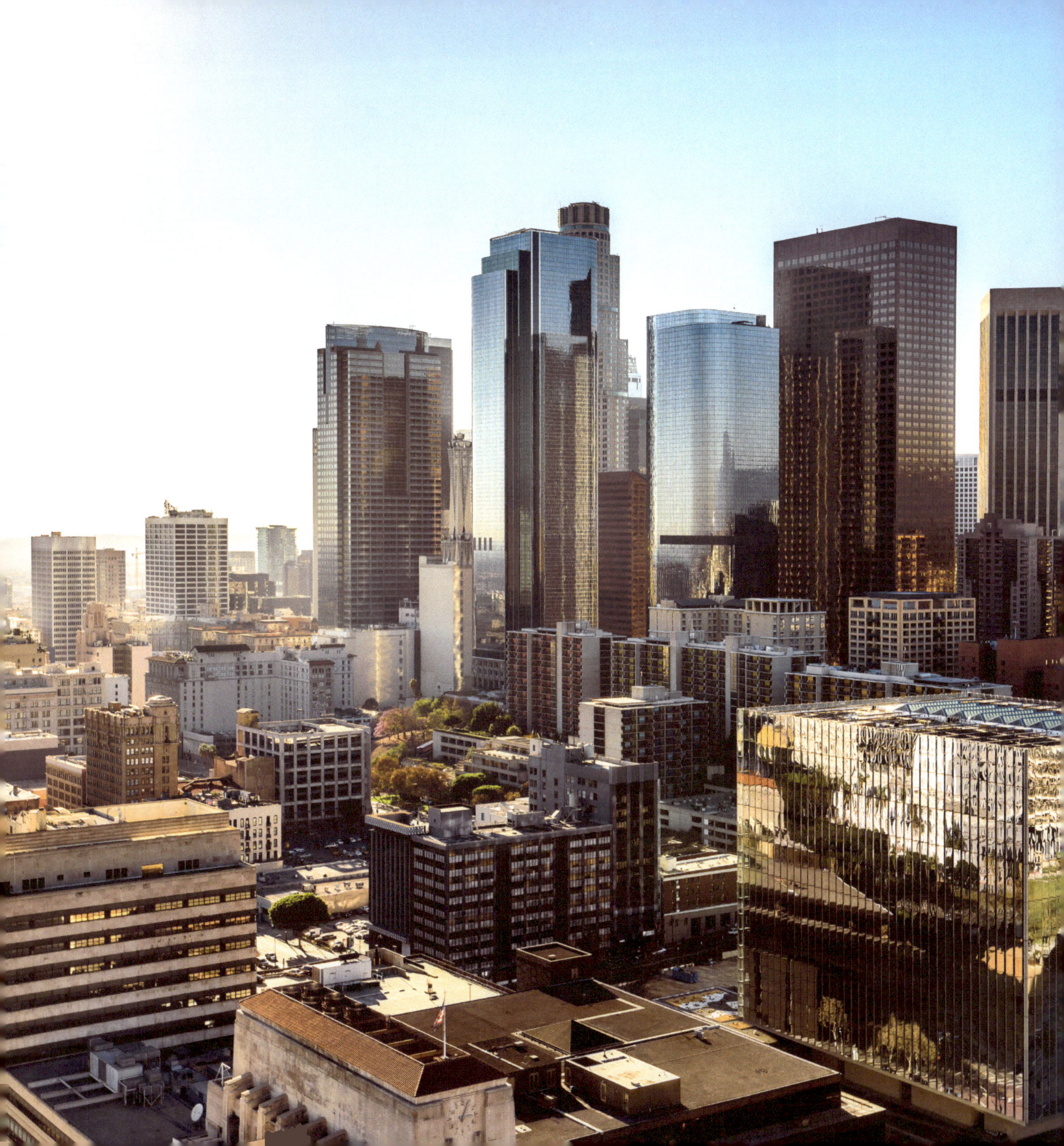

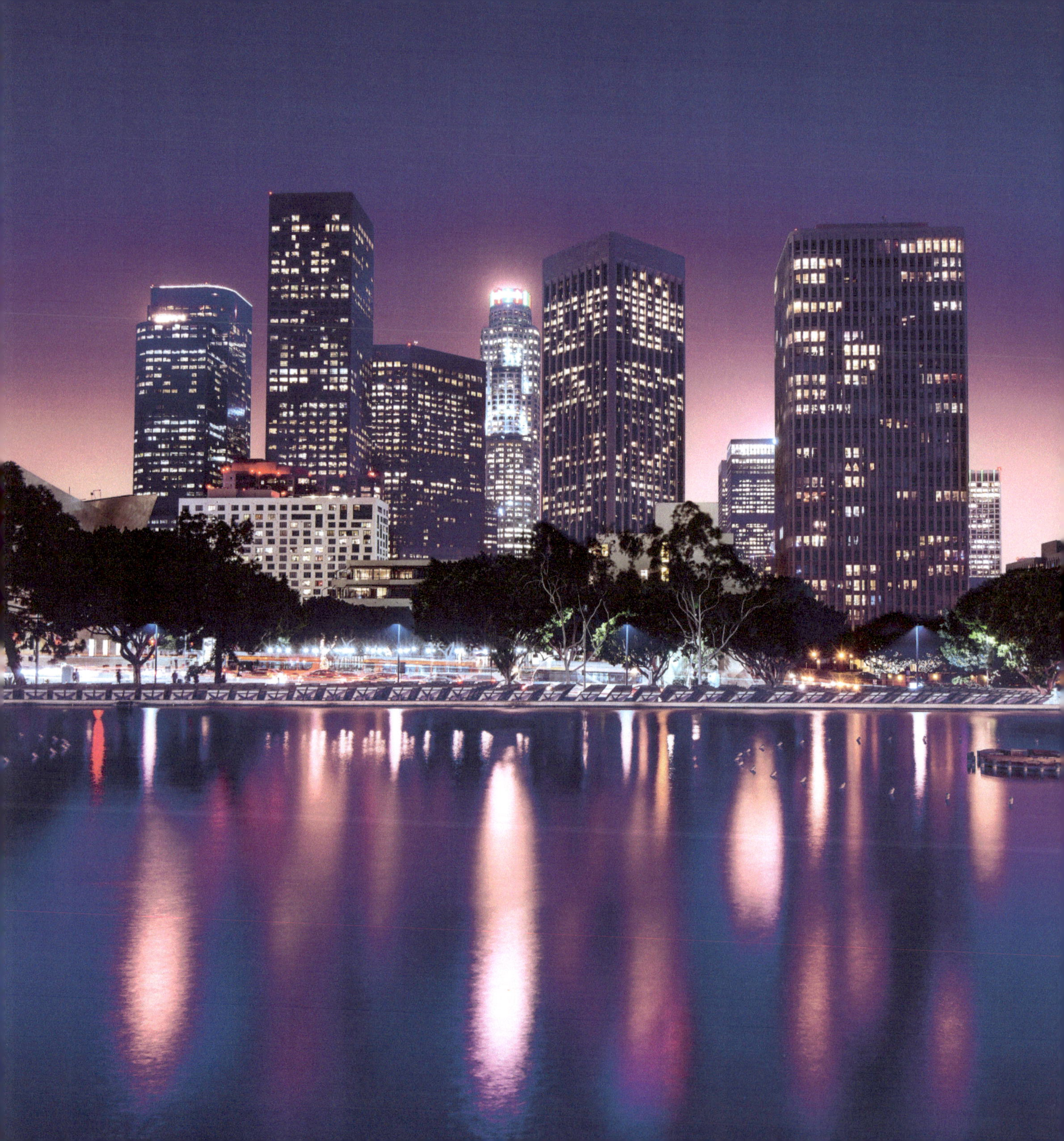

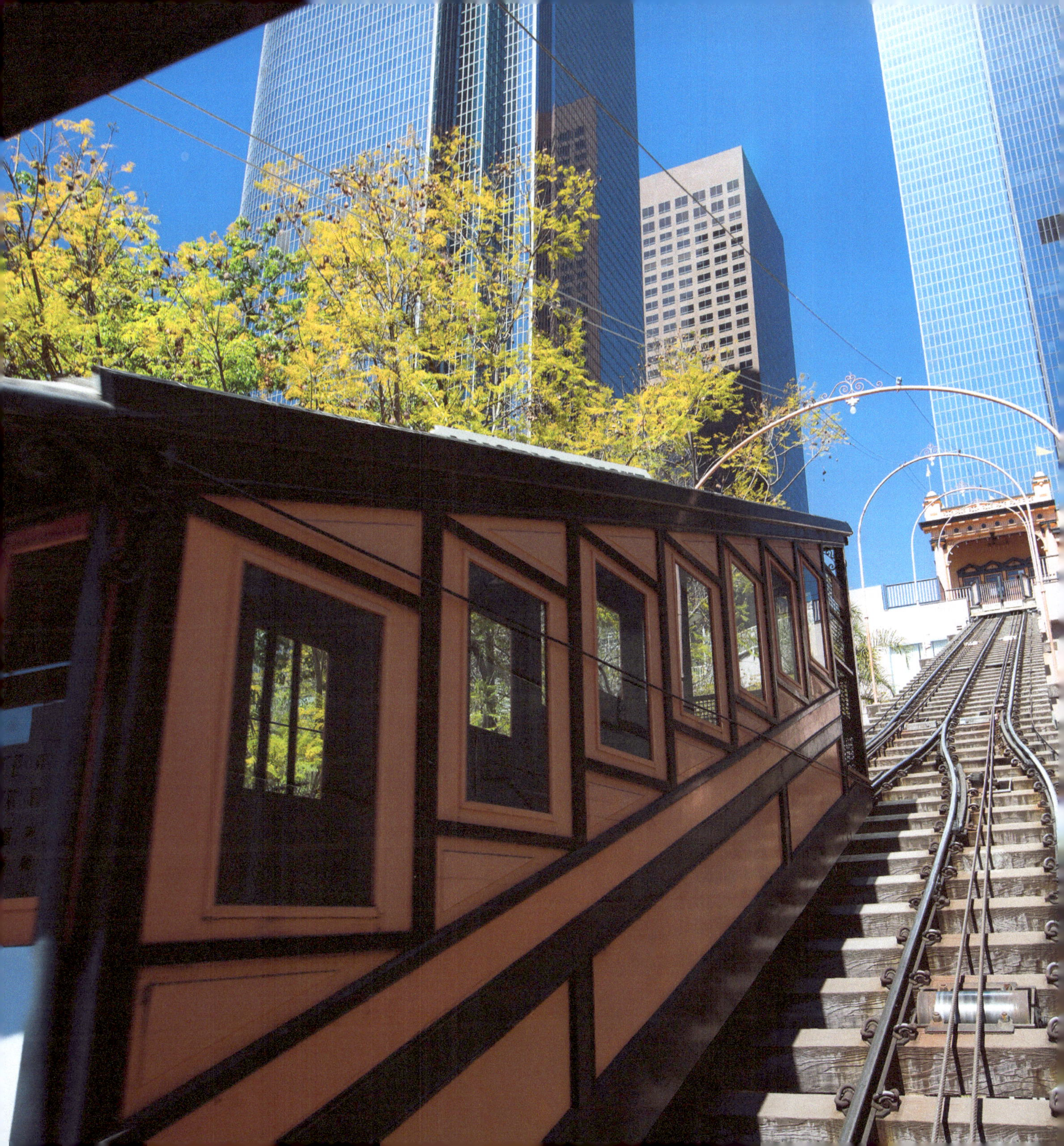

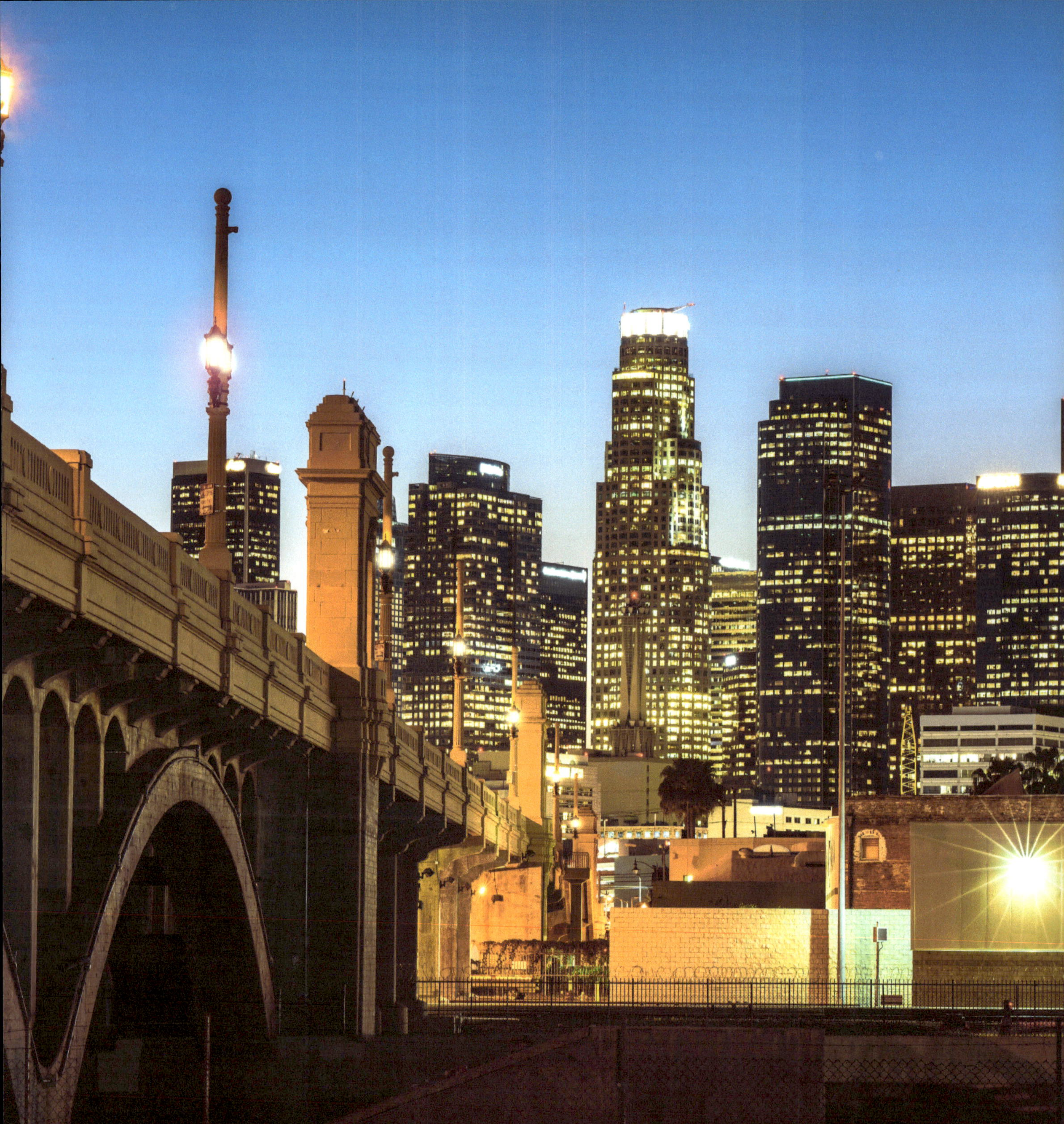

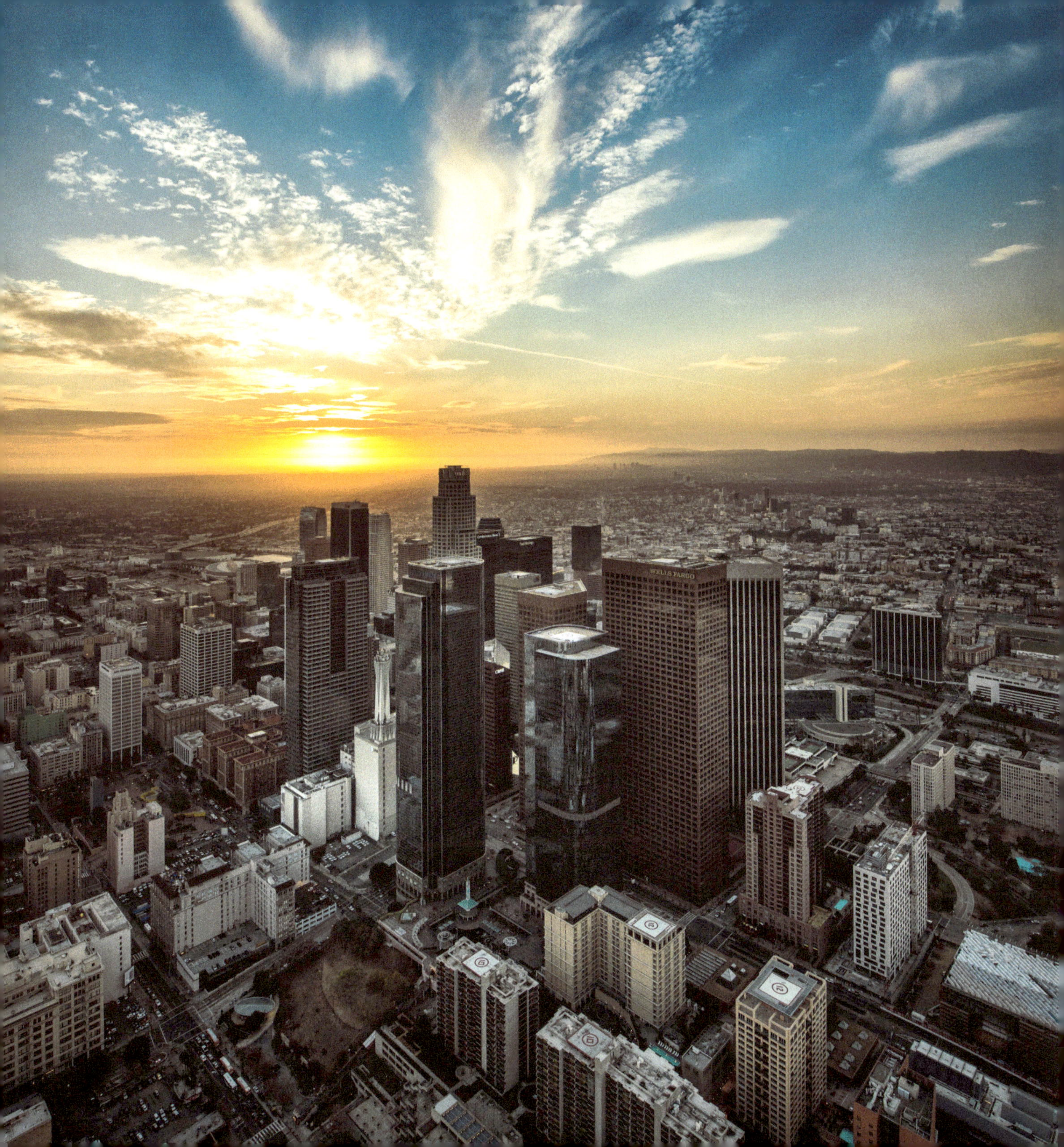

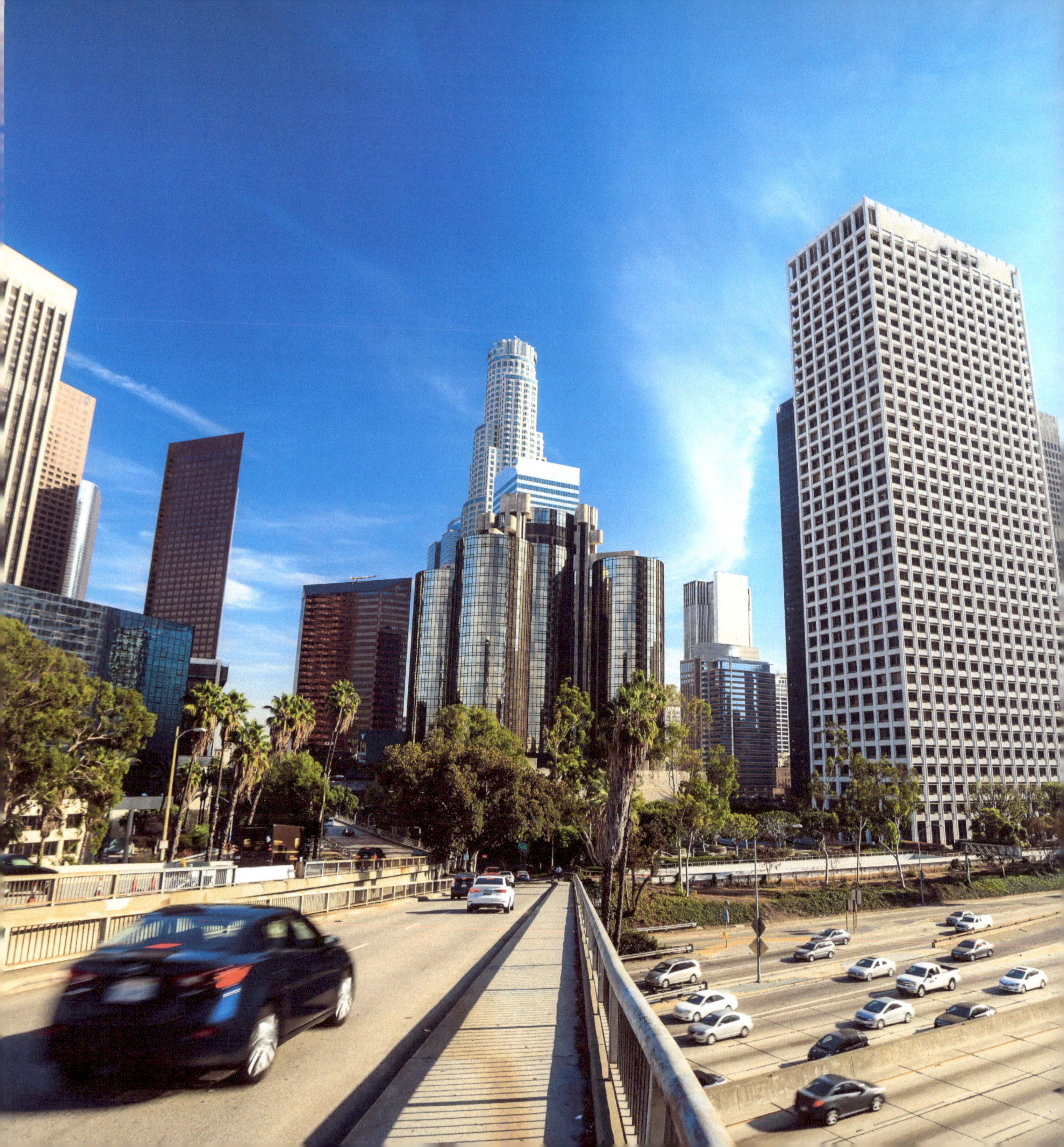

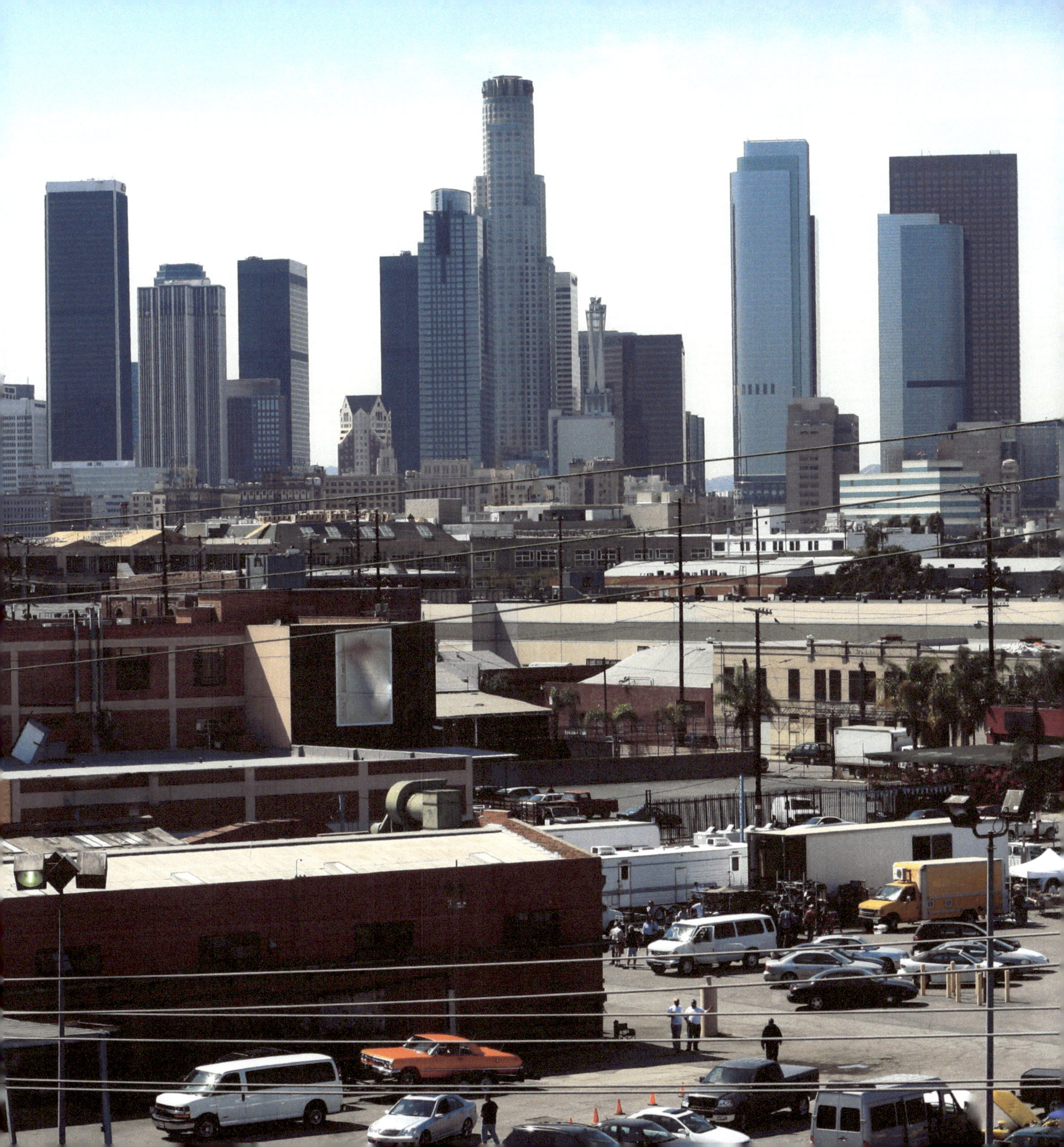

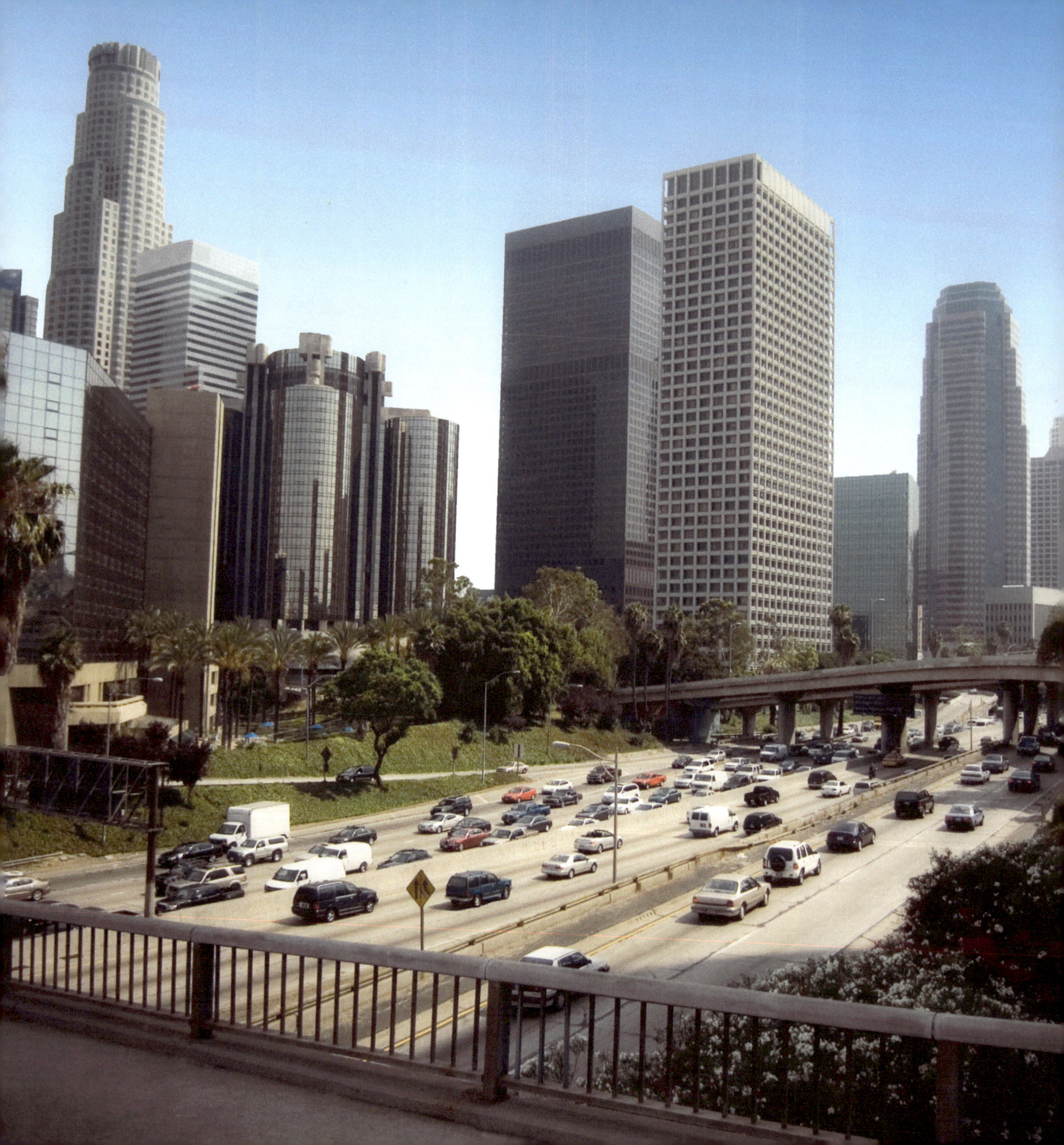

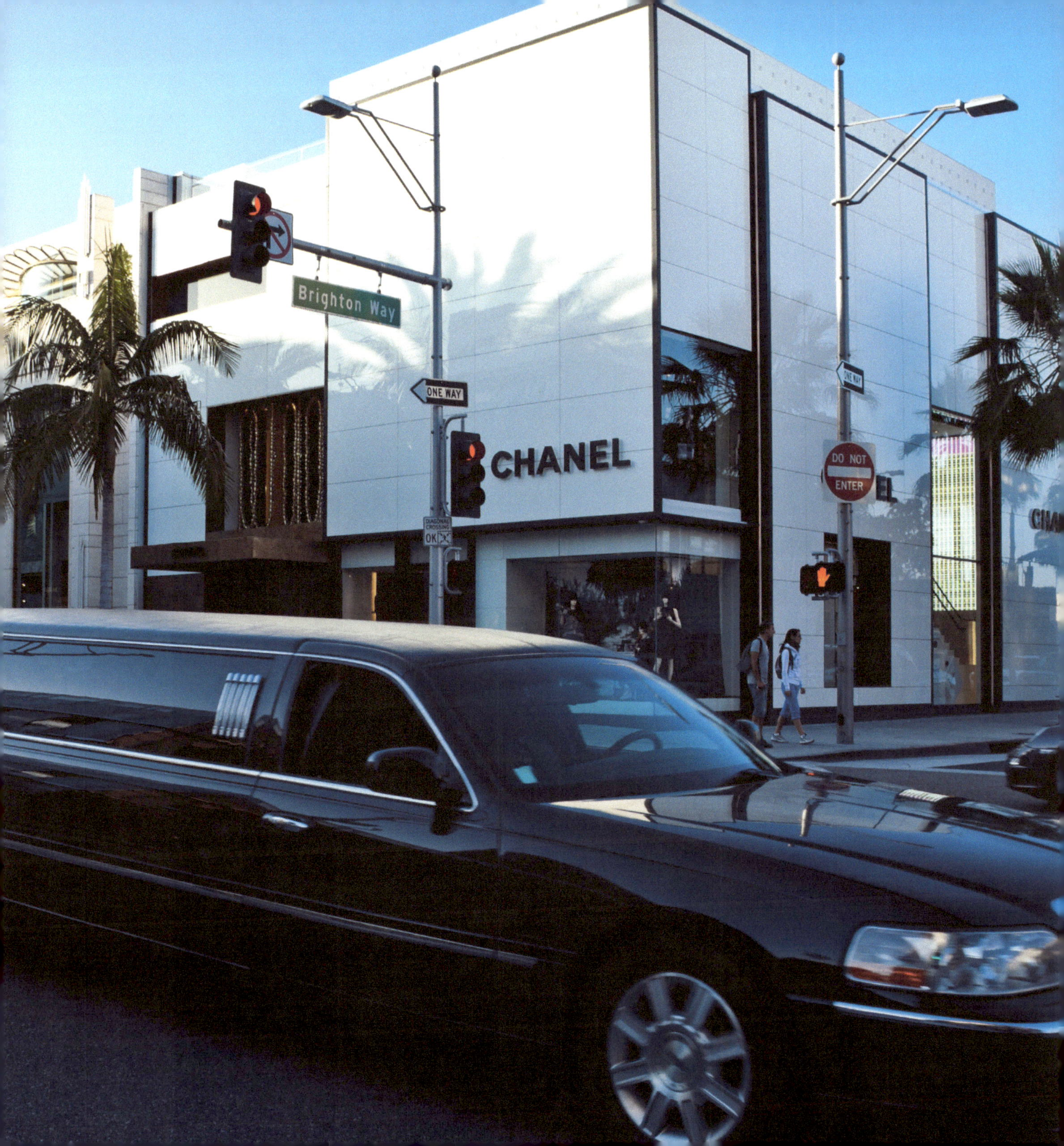

Brighton Way
ONE WAY
ONE WAY
CHANEL
CHANEL
DO NOT ENTER
DIAGONAL CROSSING OK

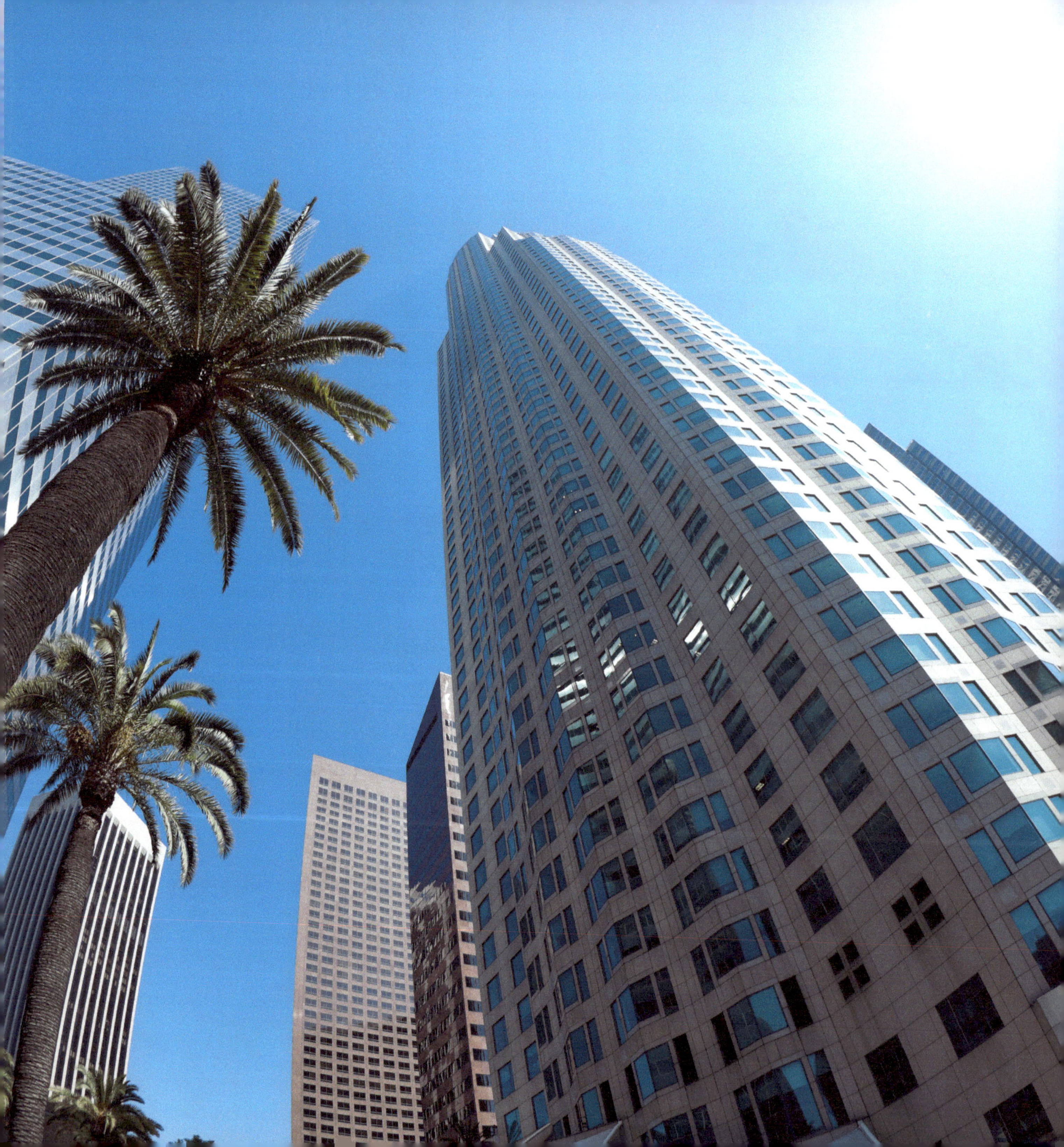

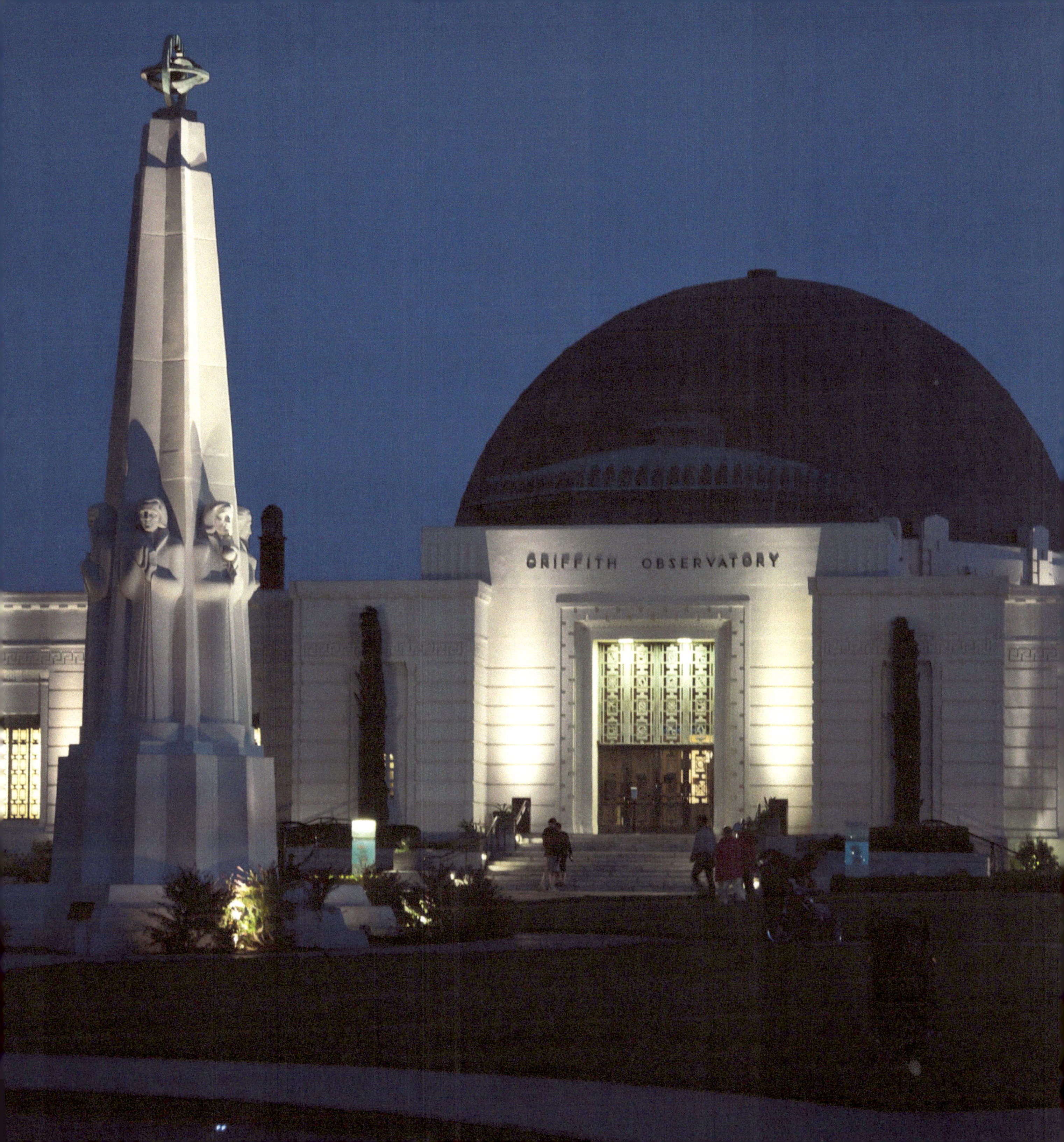
GRIFFITH OBSERVATORY

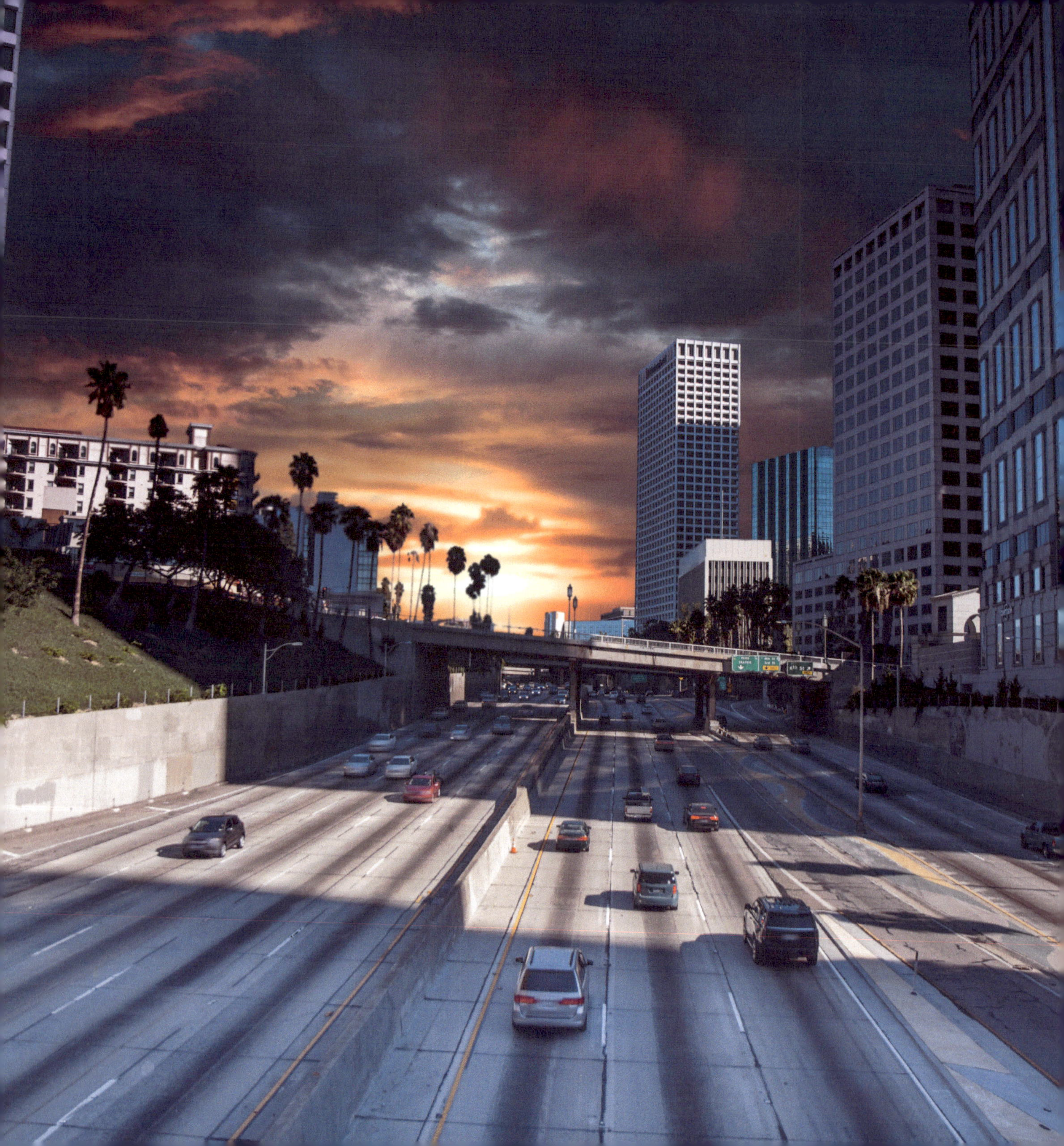

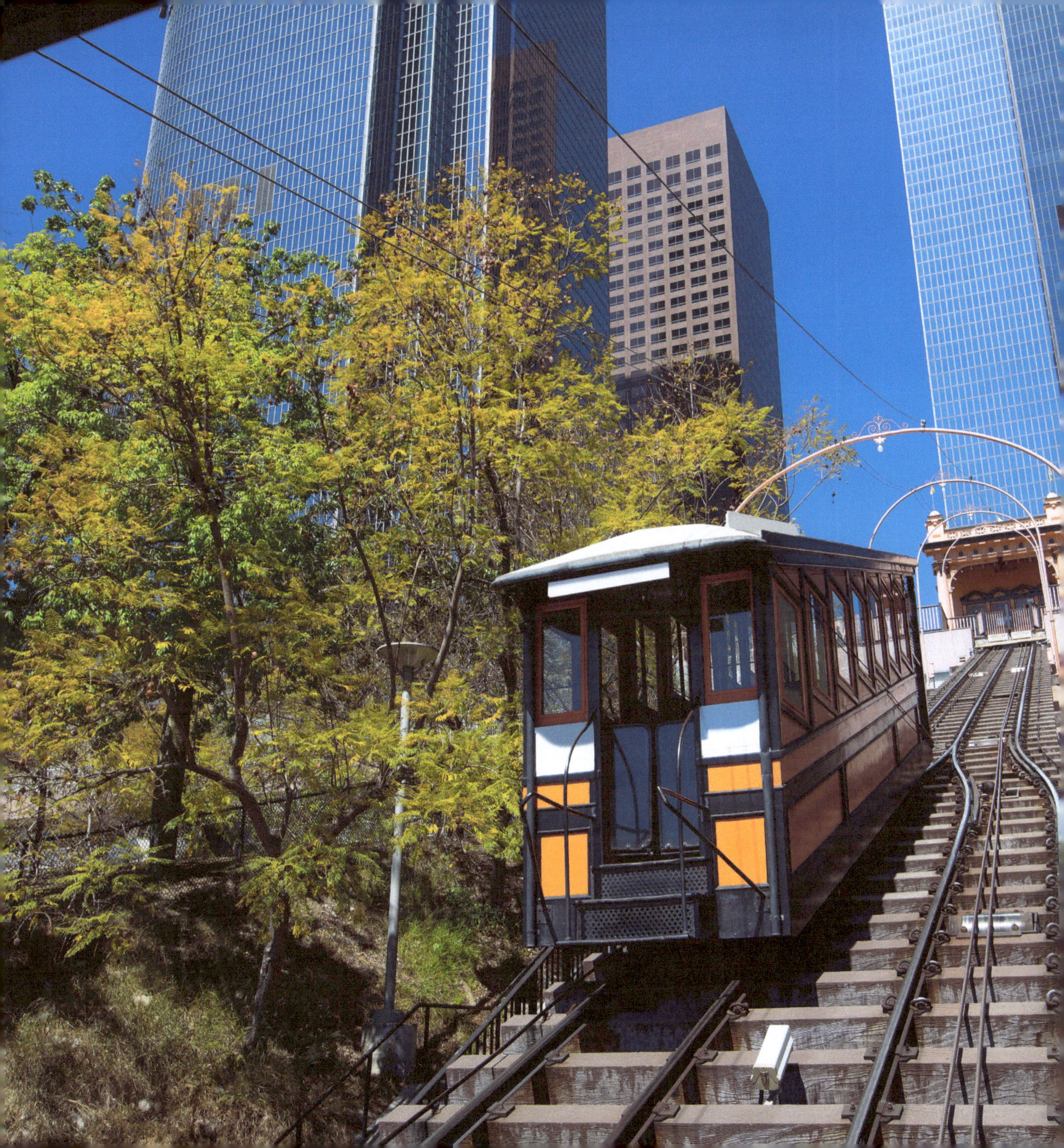

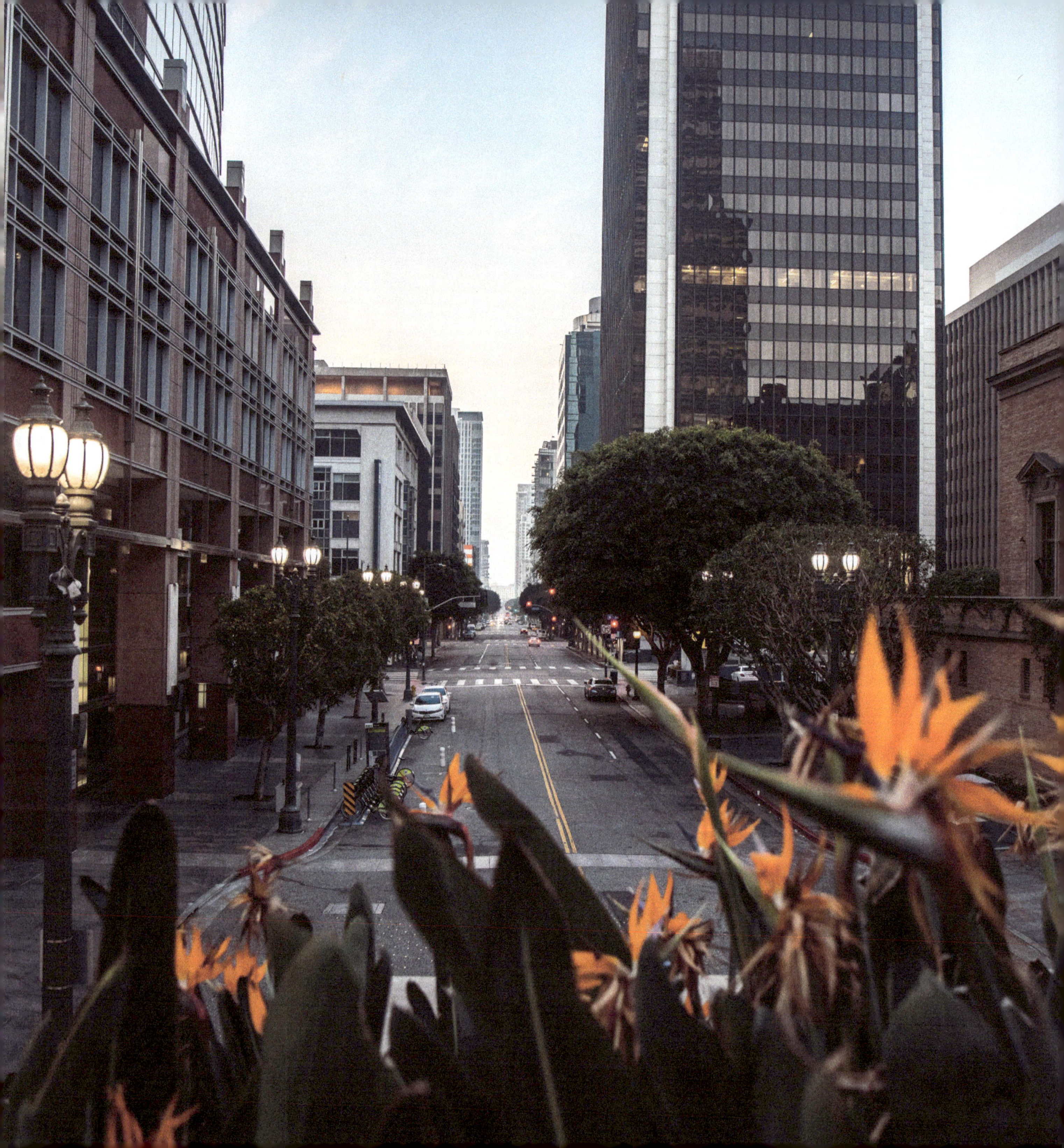

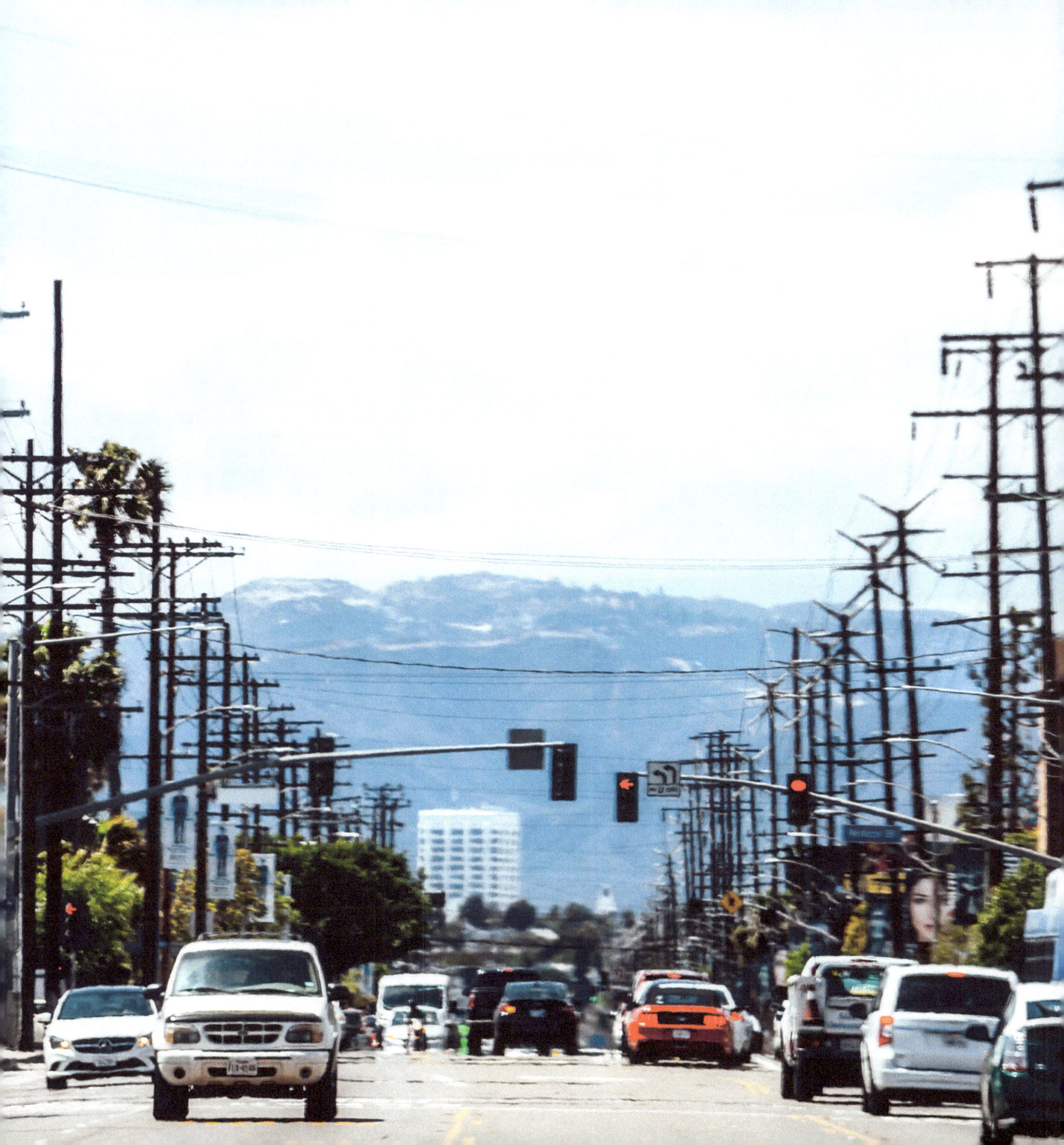

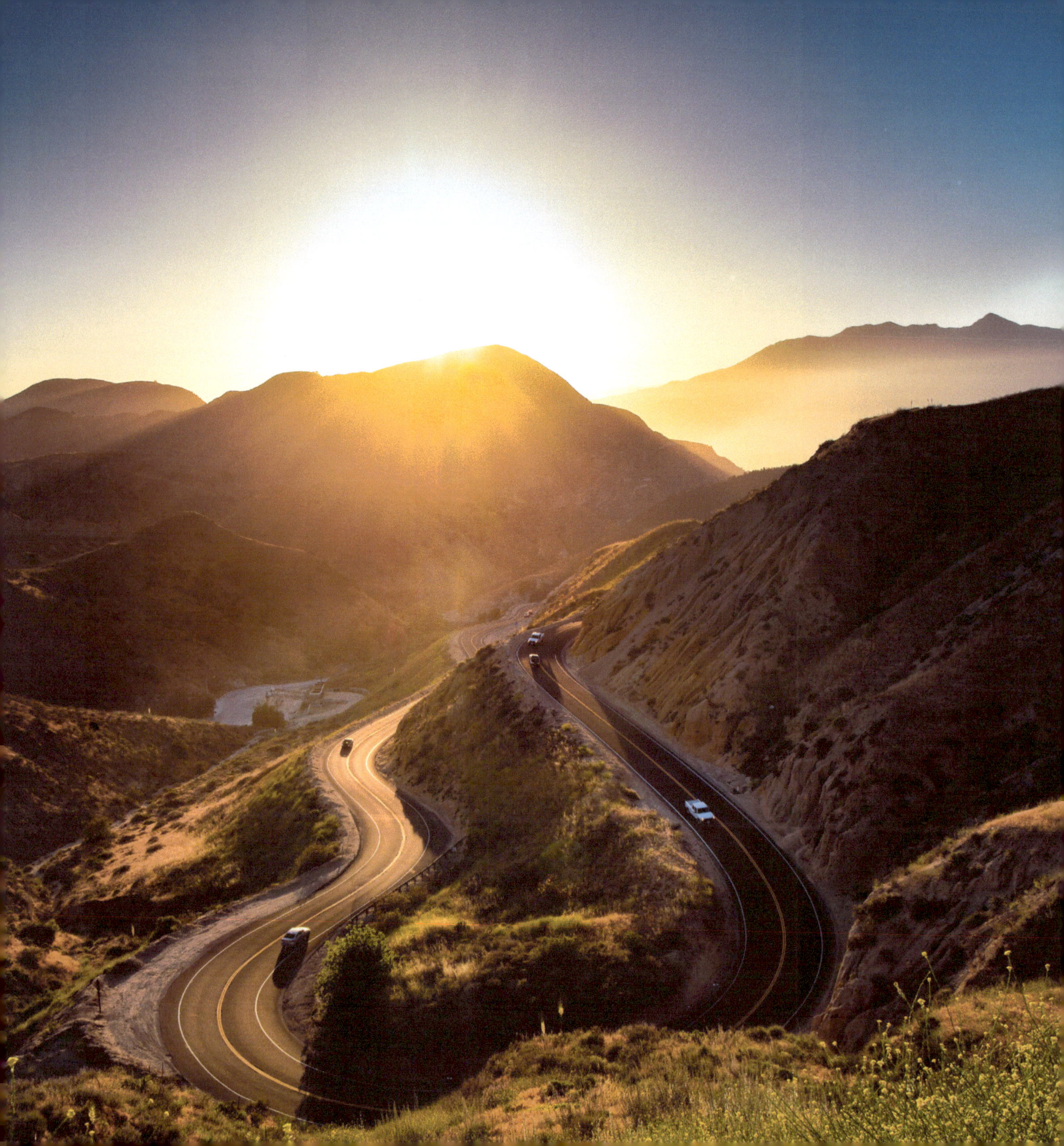

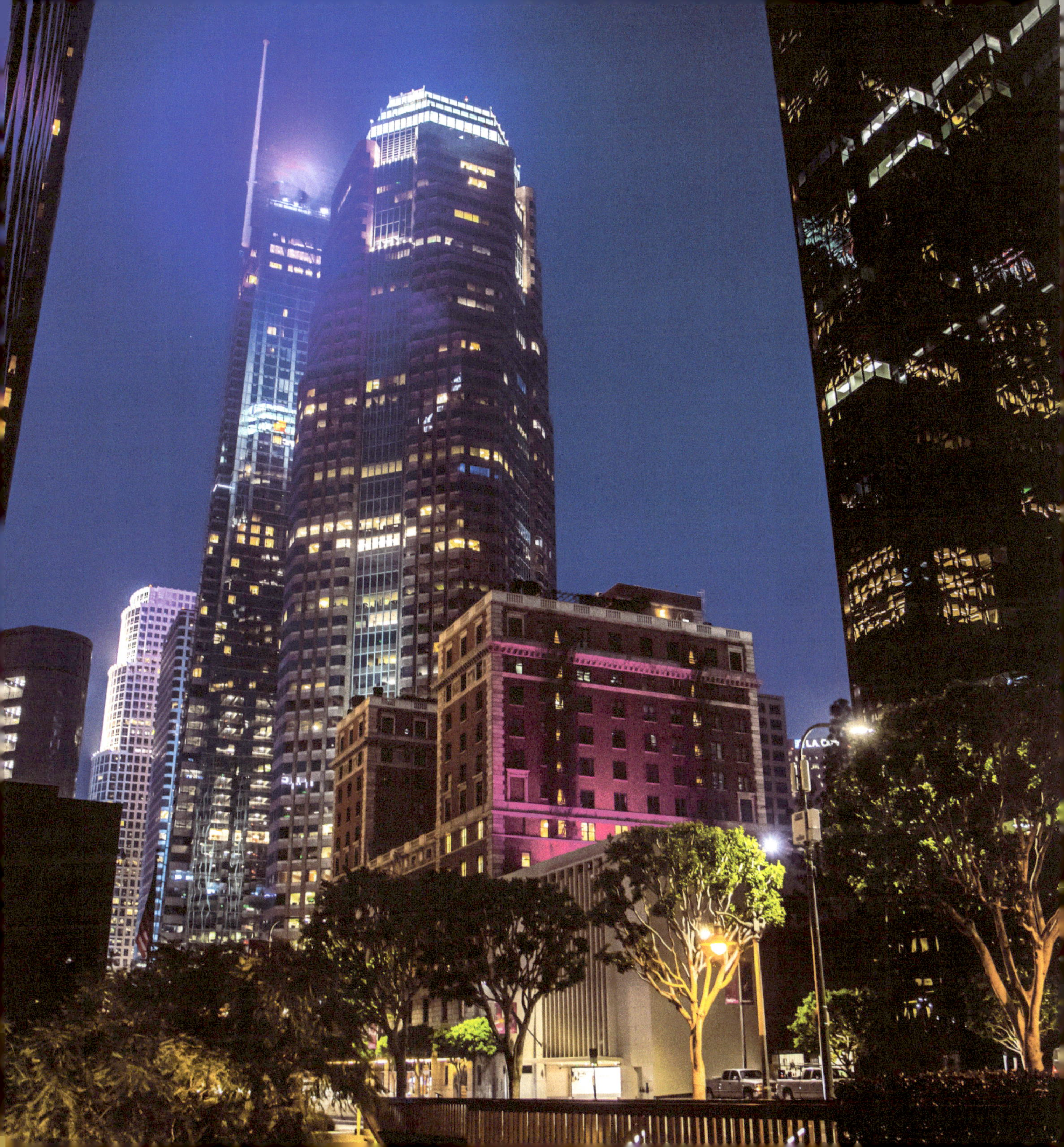

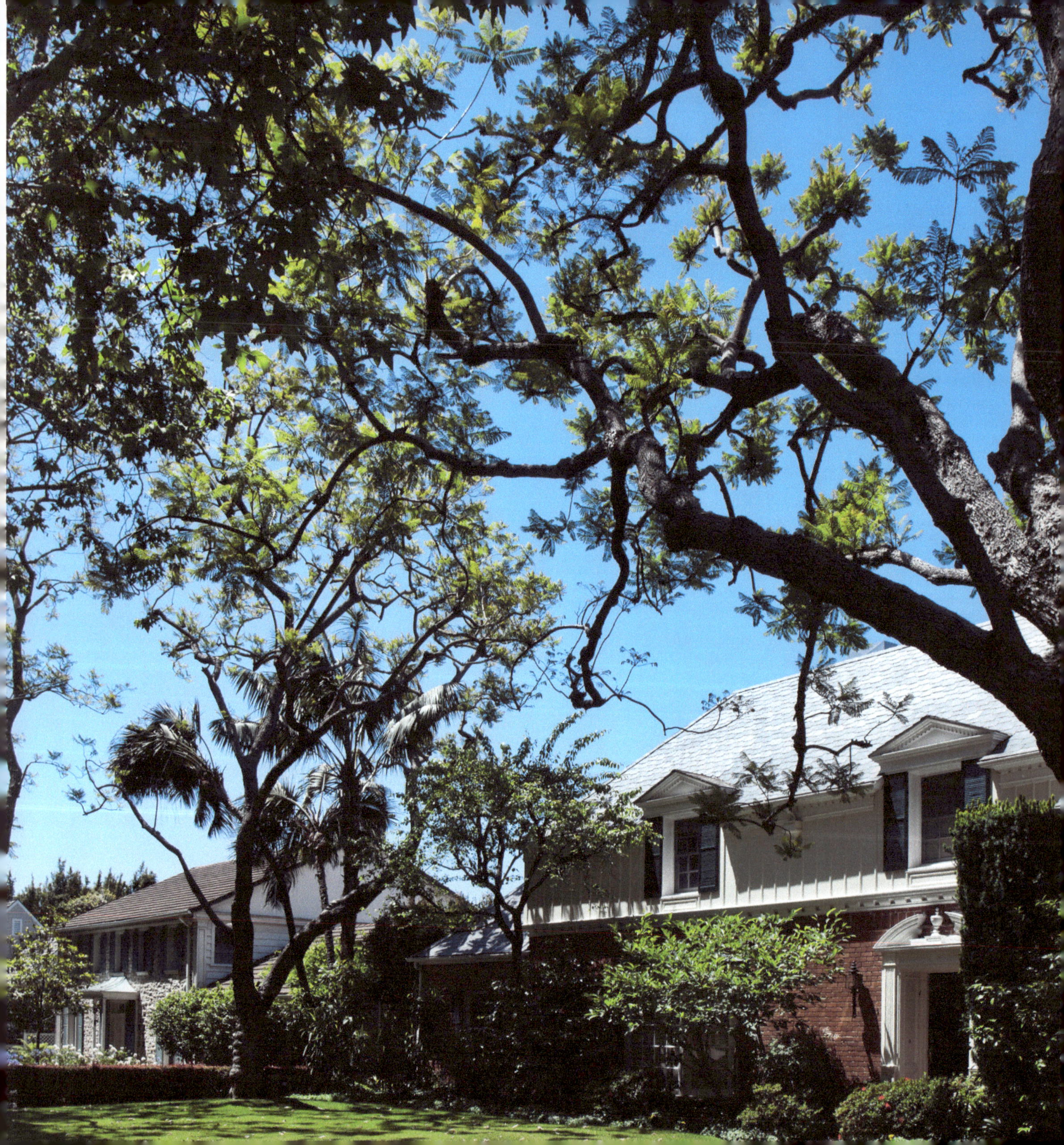

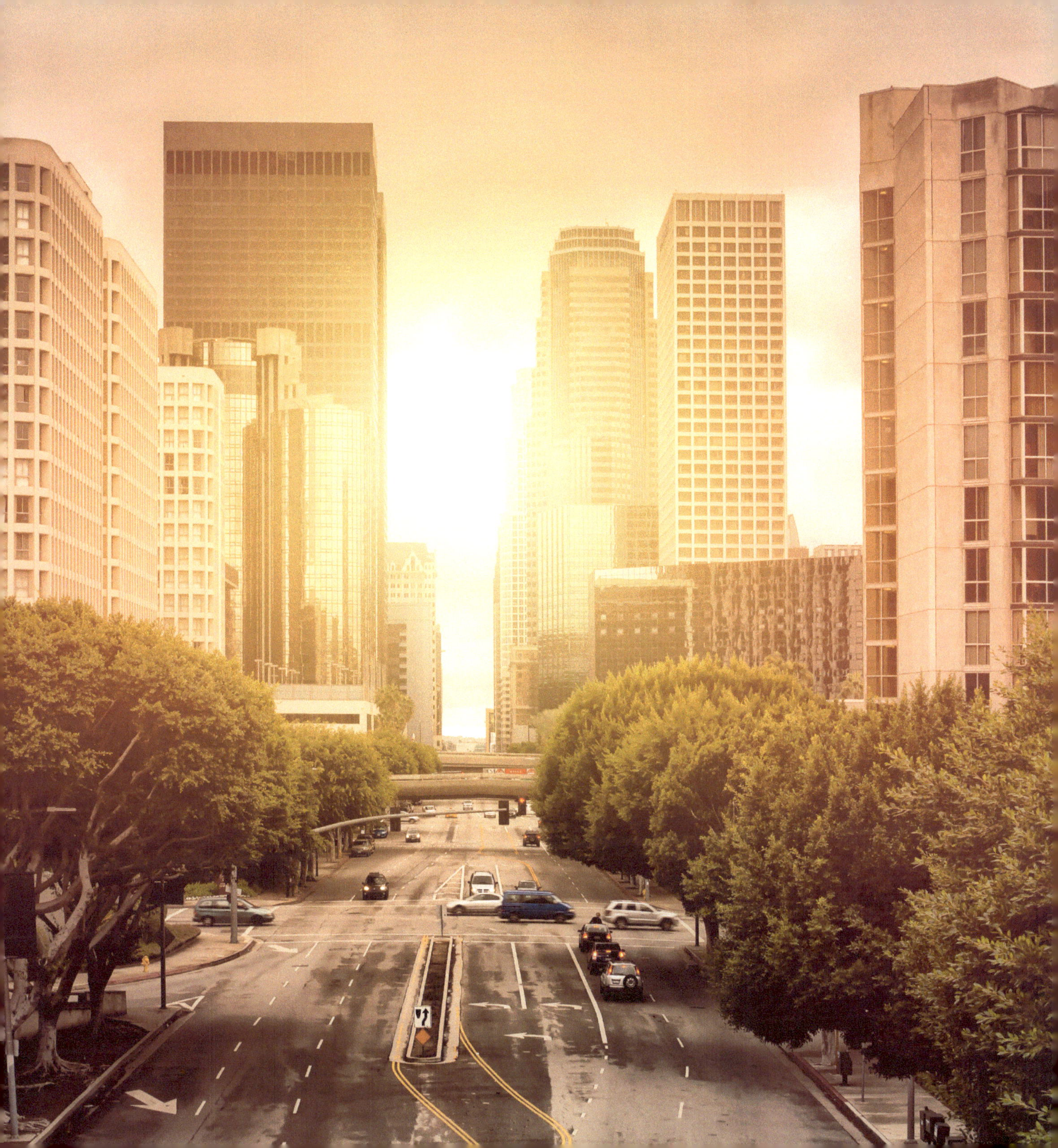

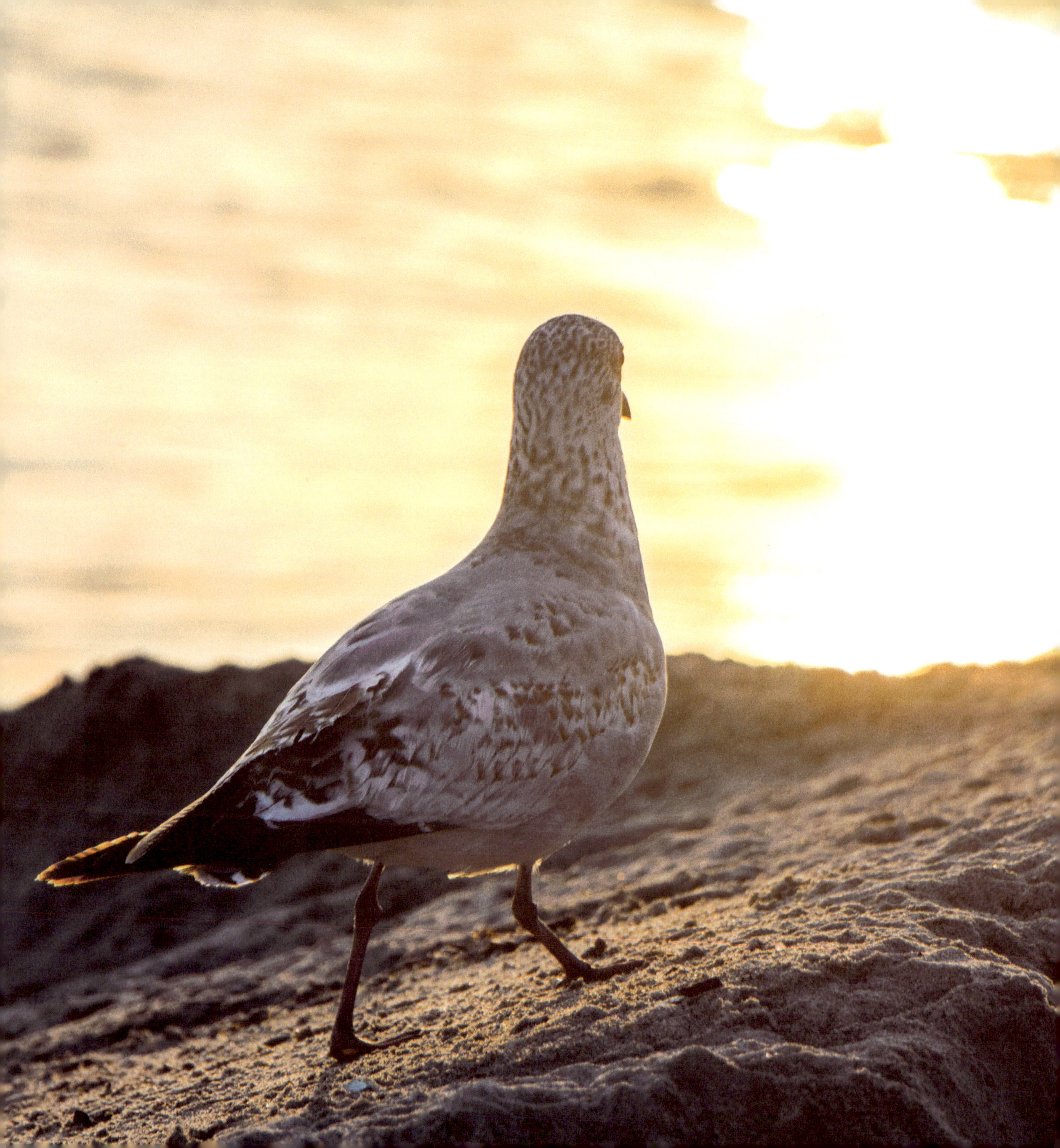

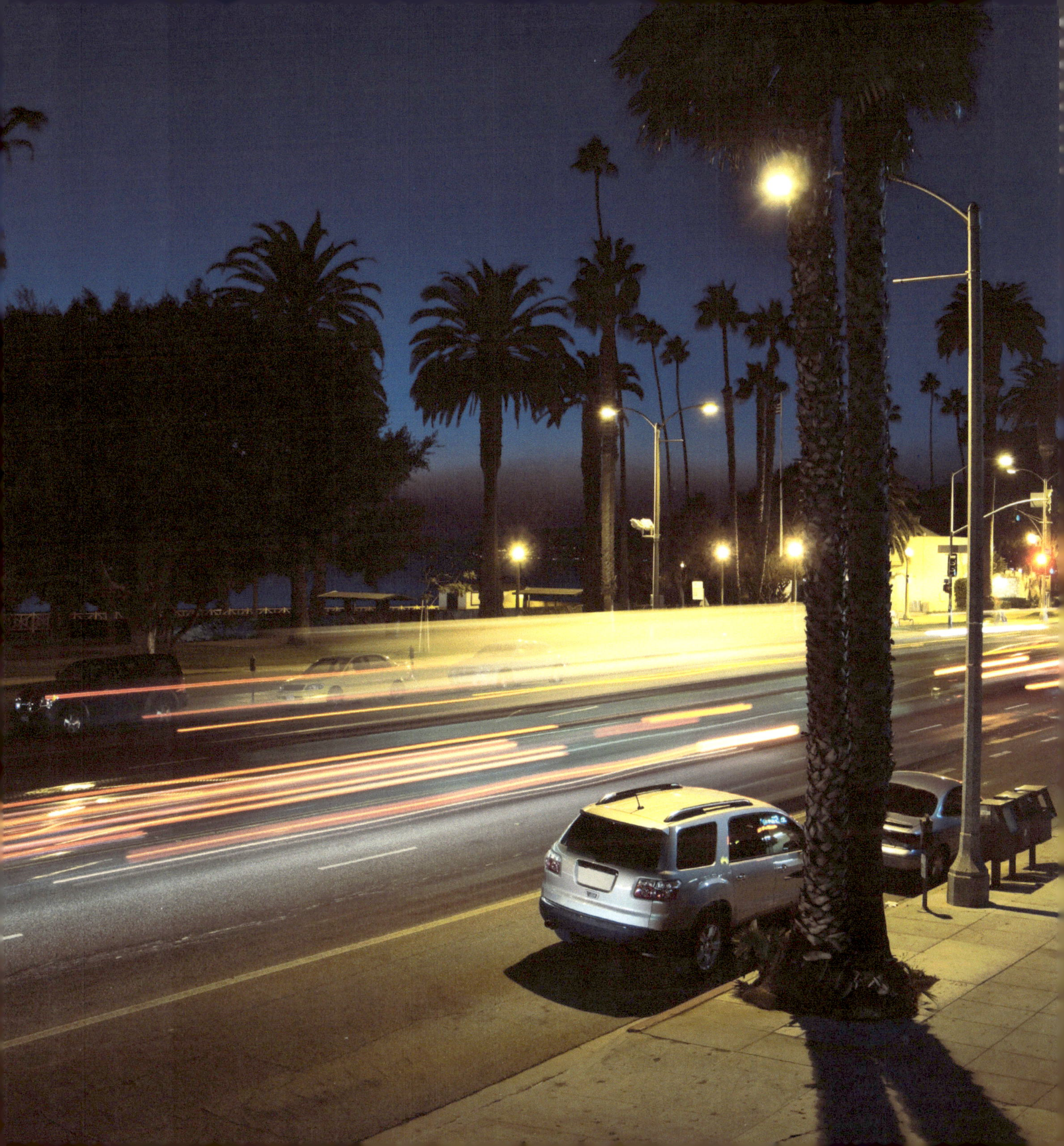

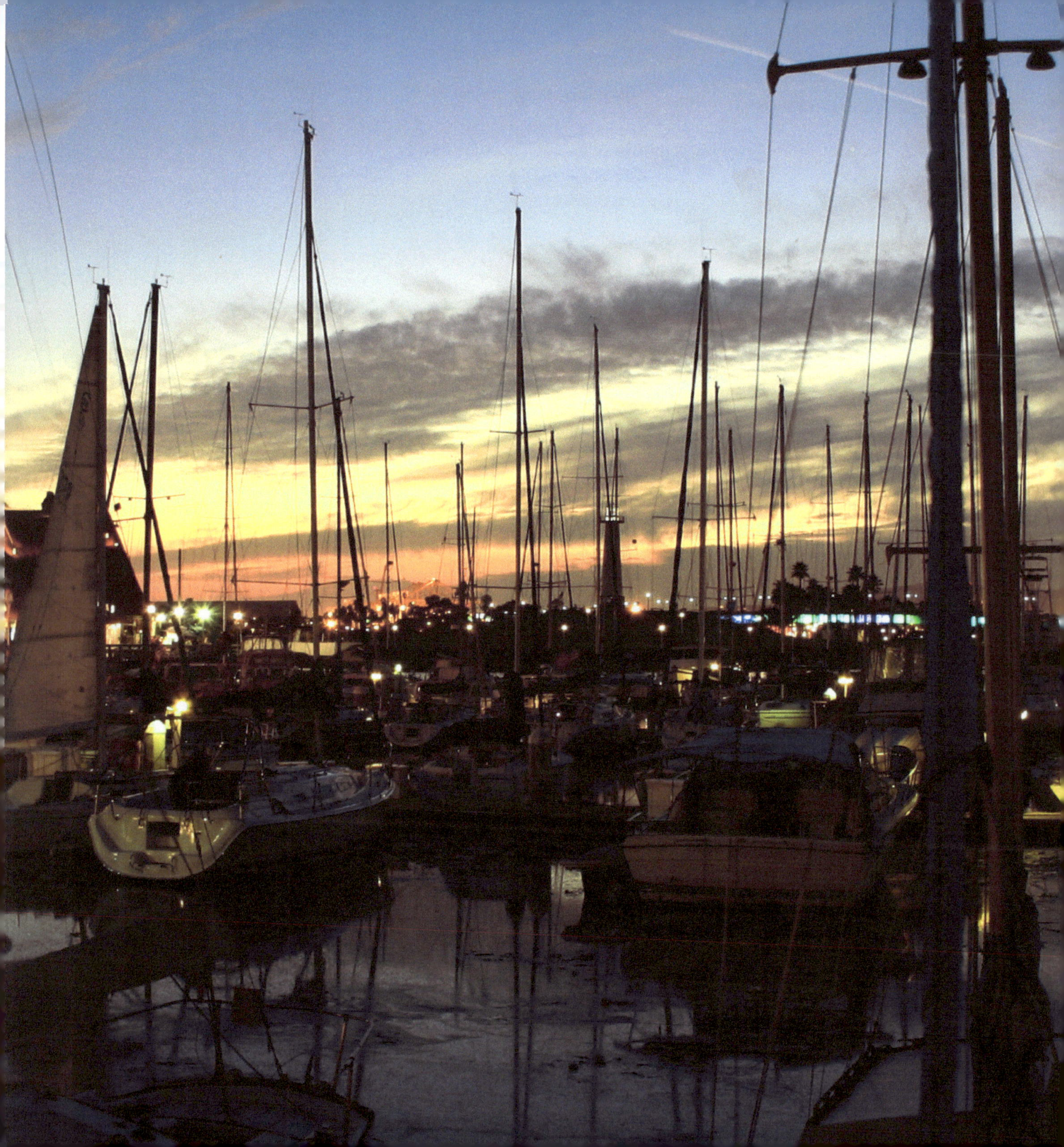

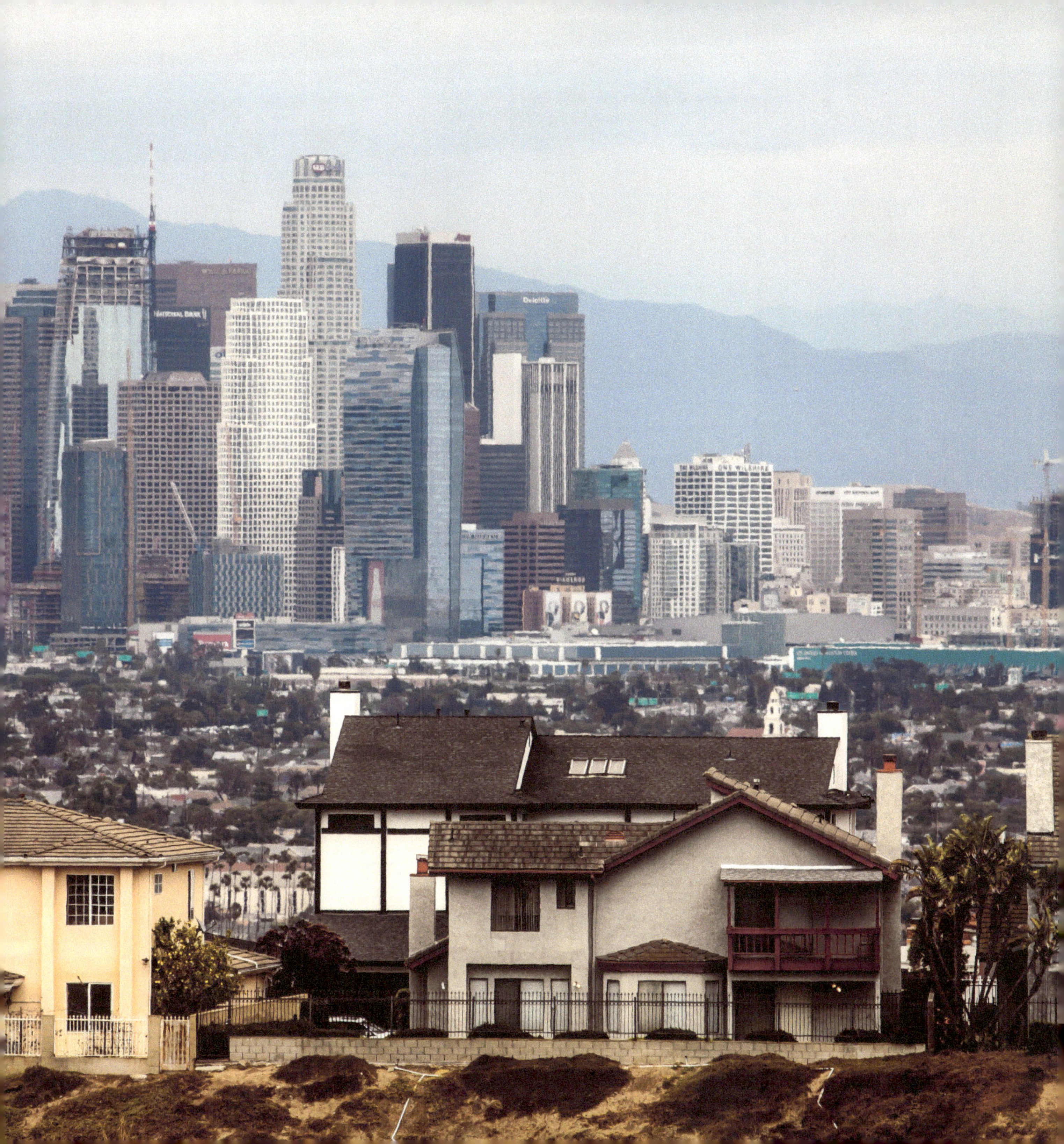

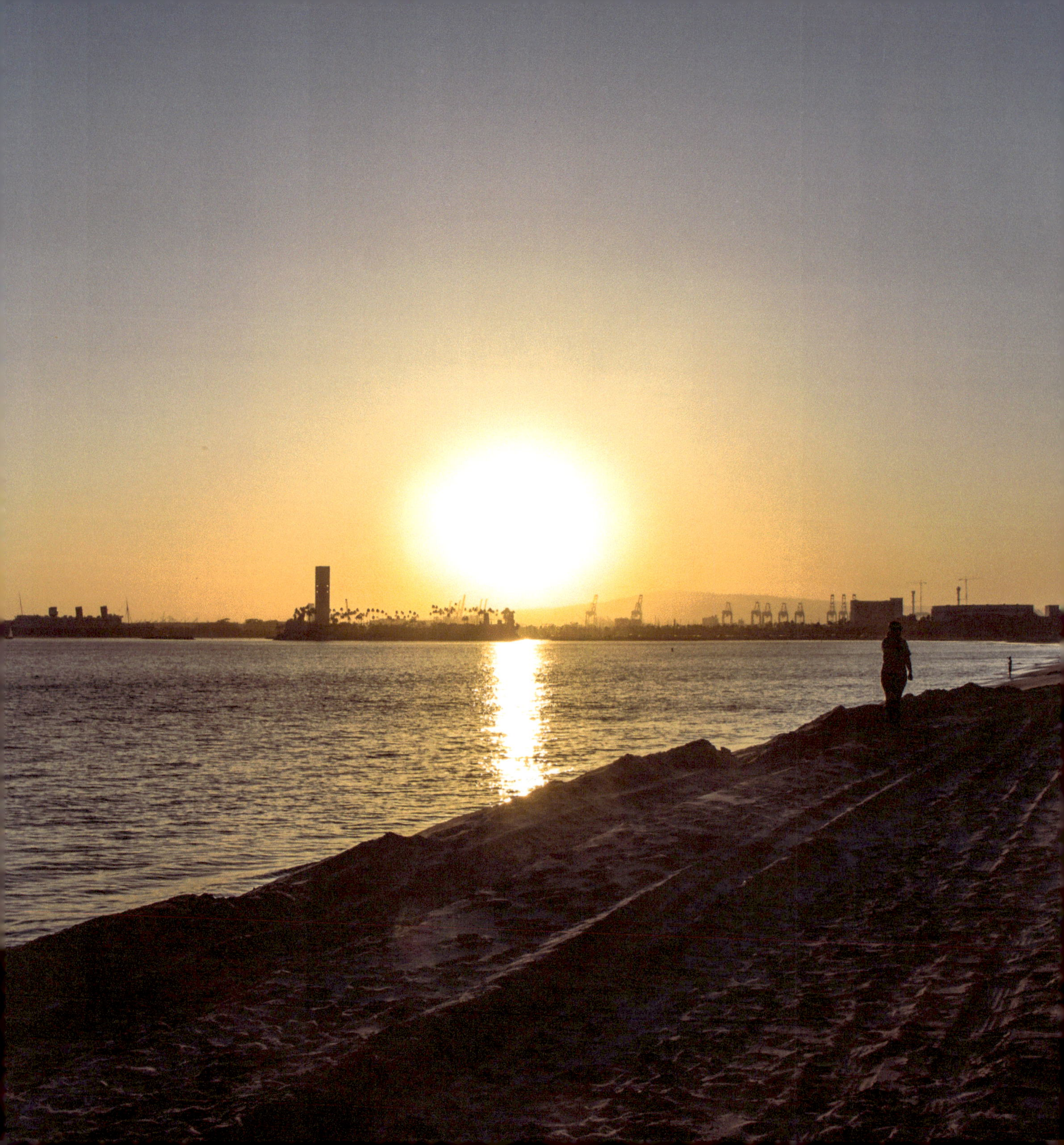

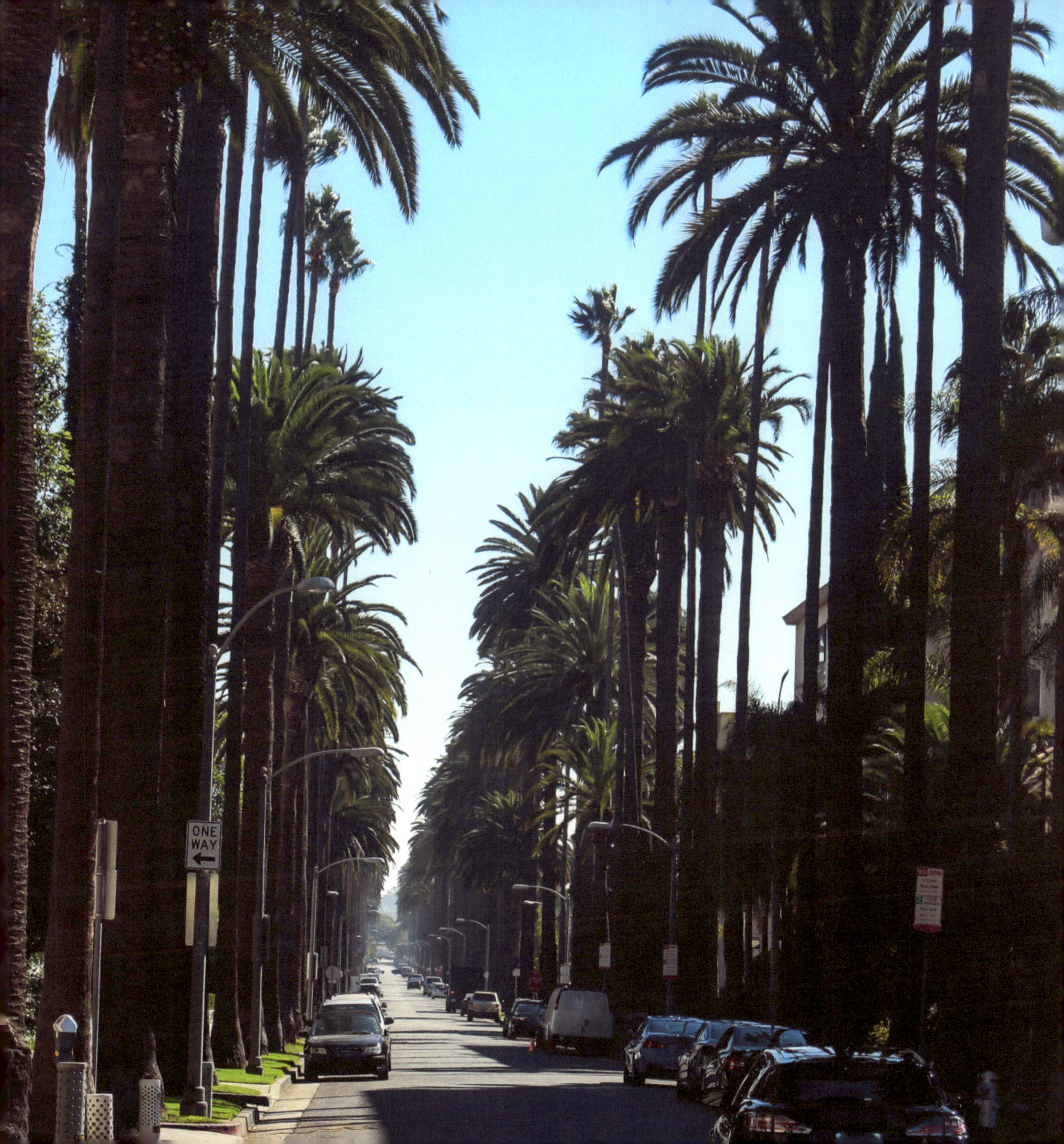

ONE
WAY

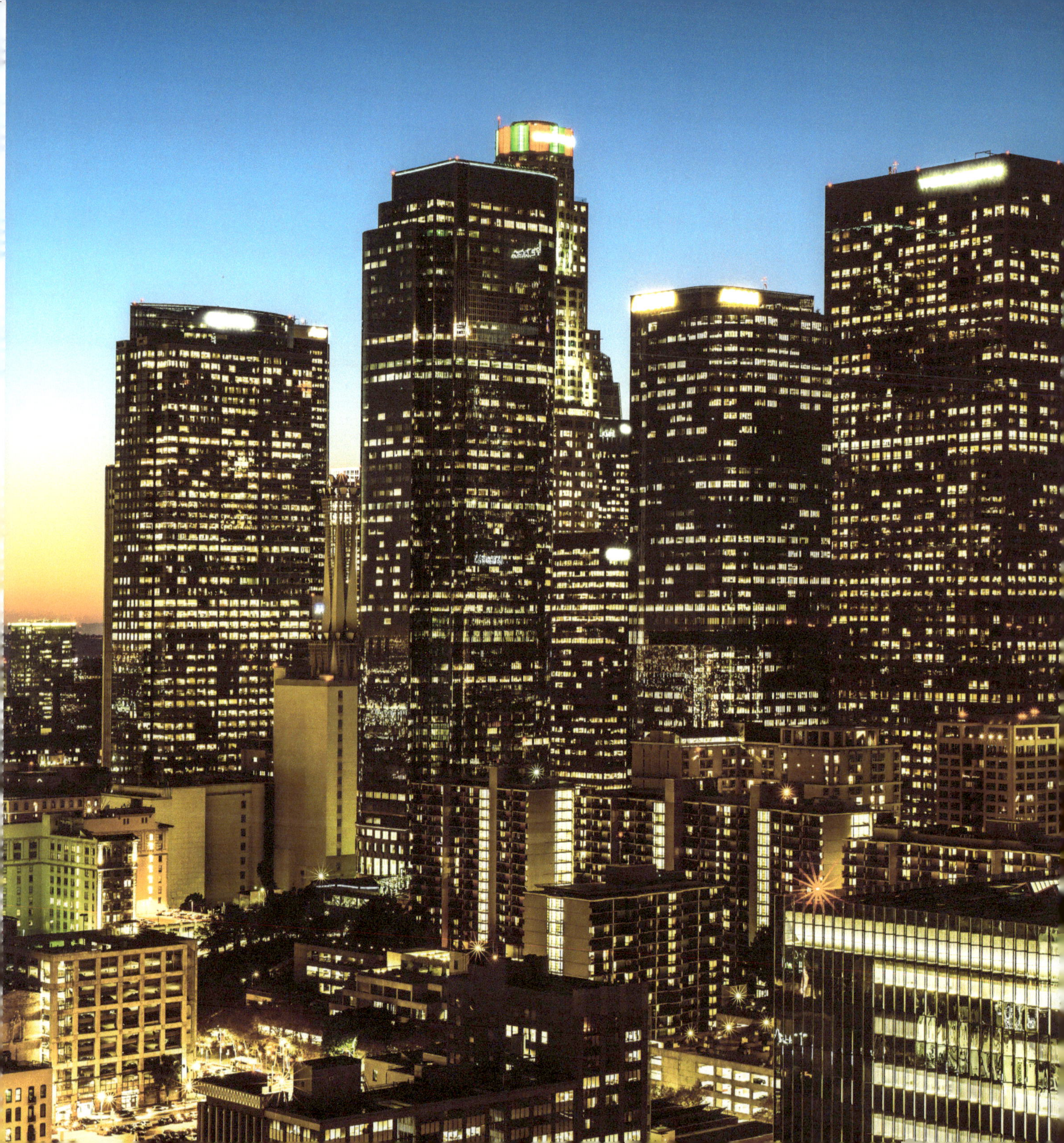

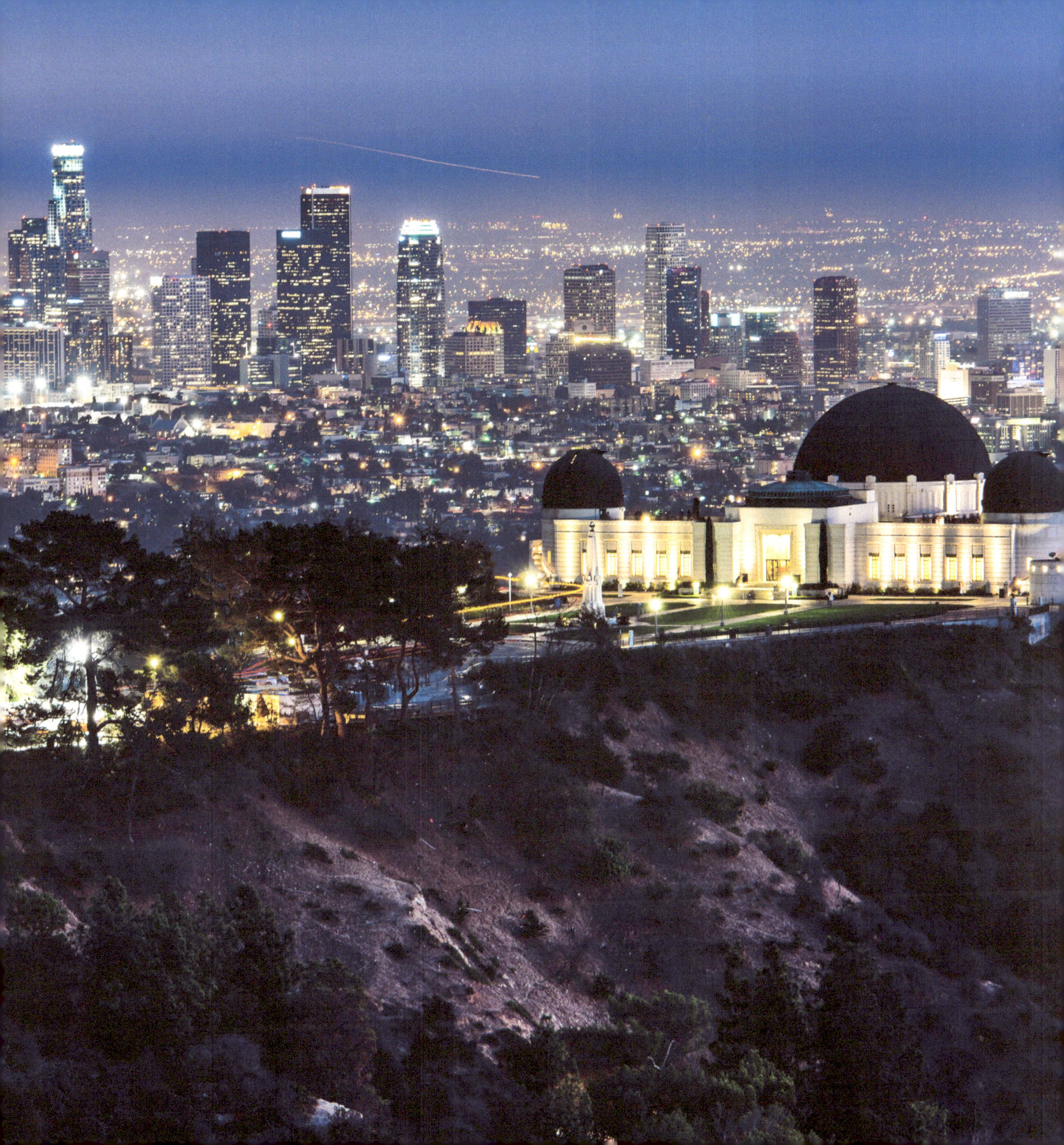

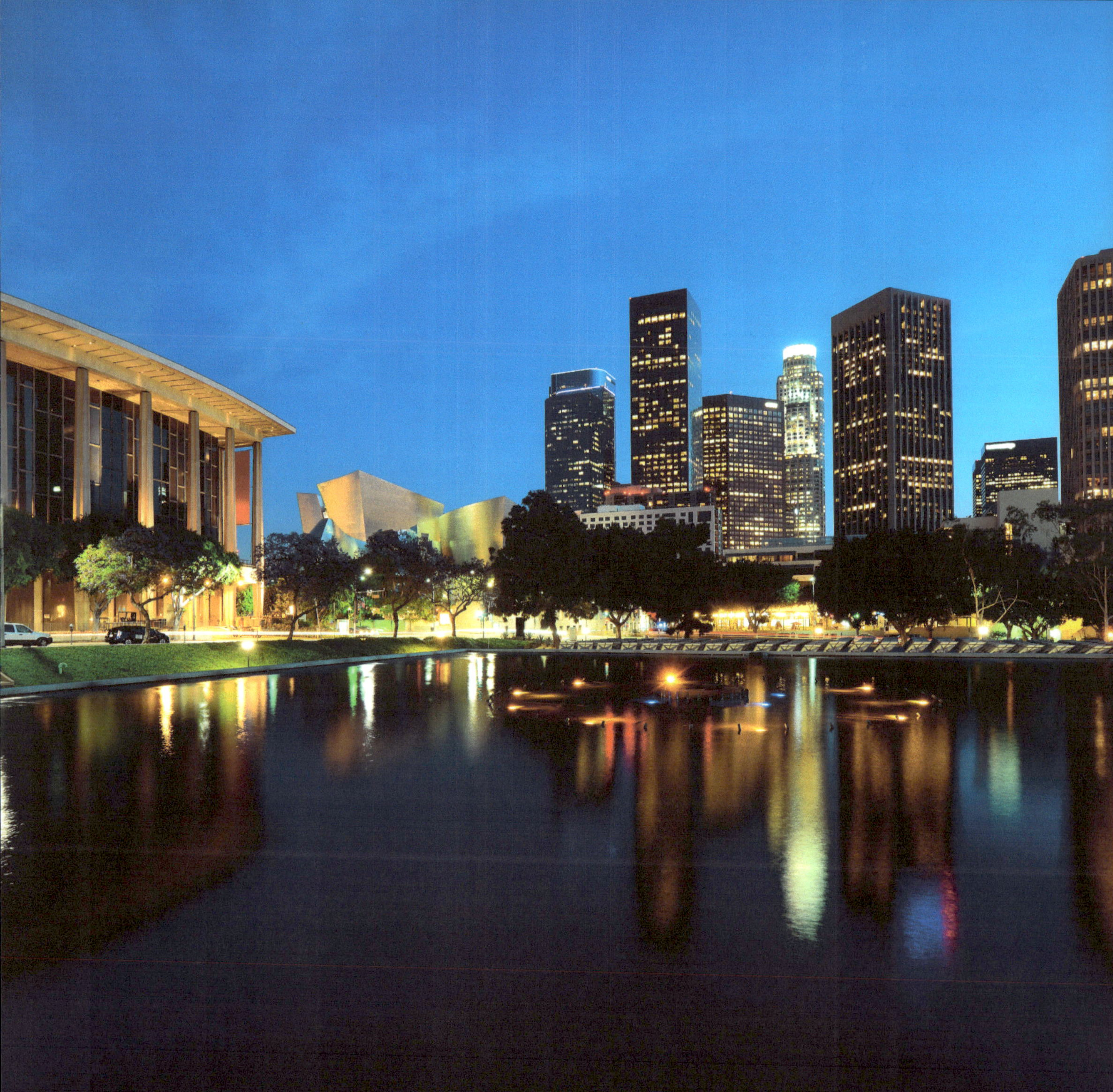

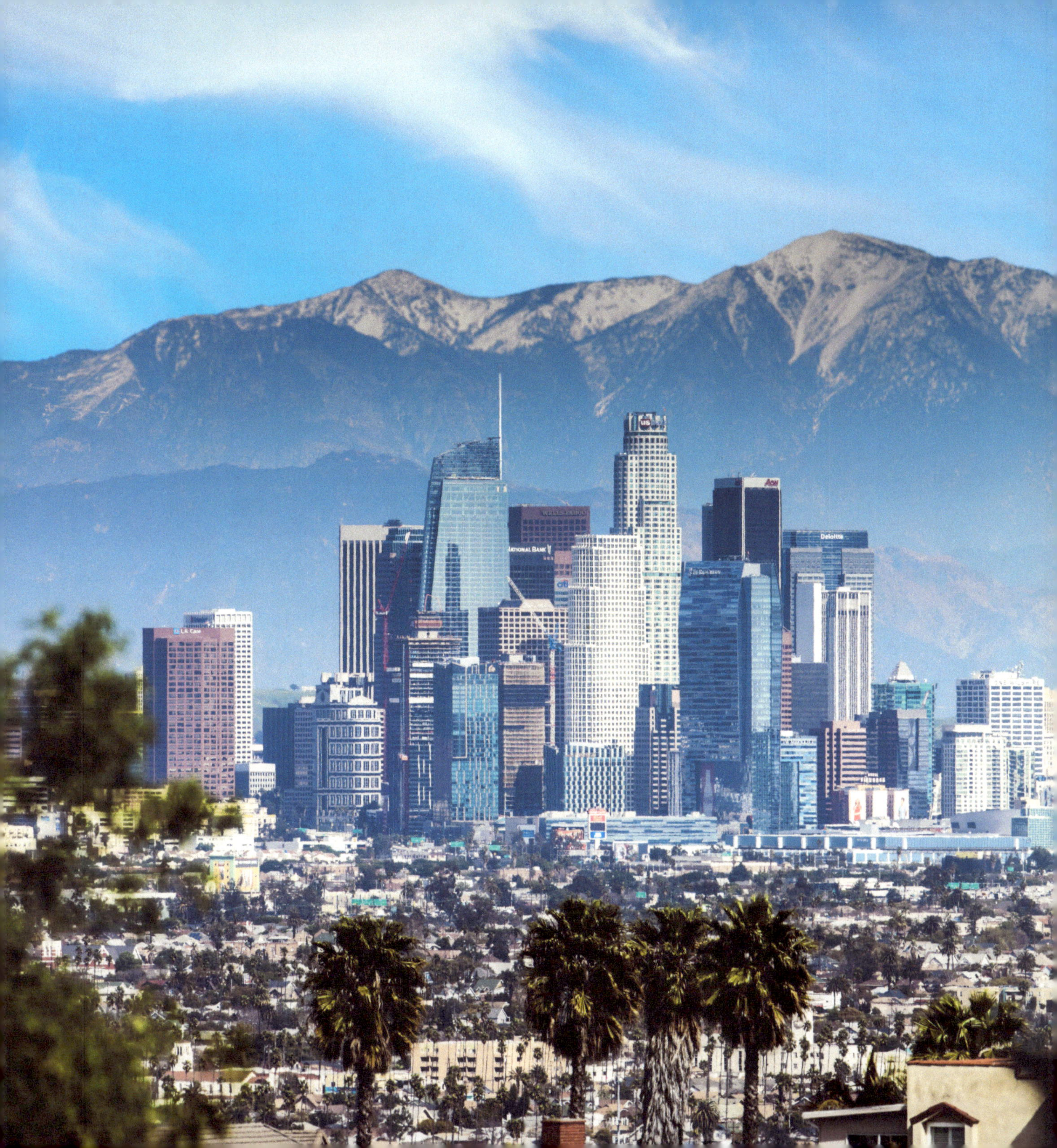

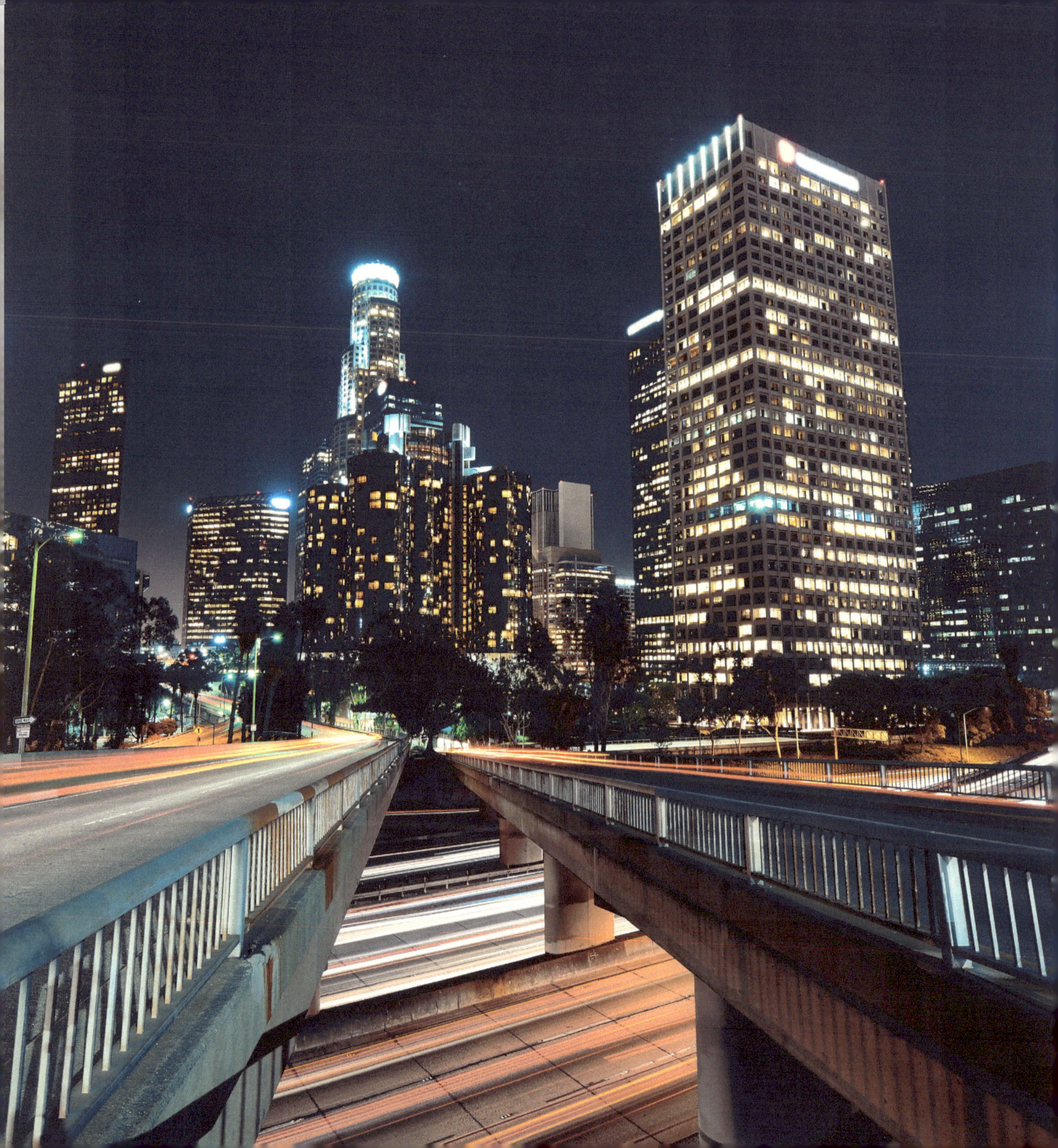

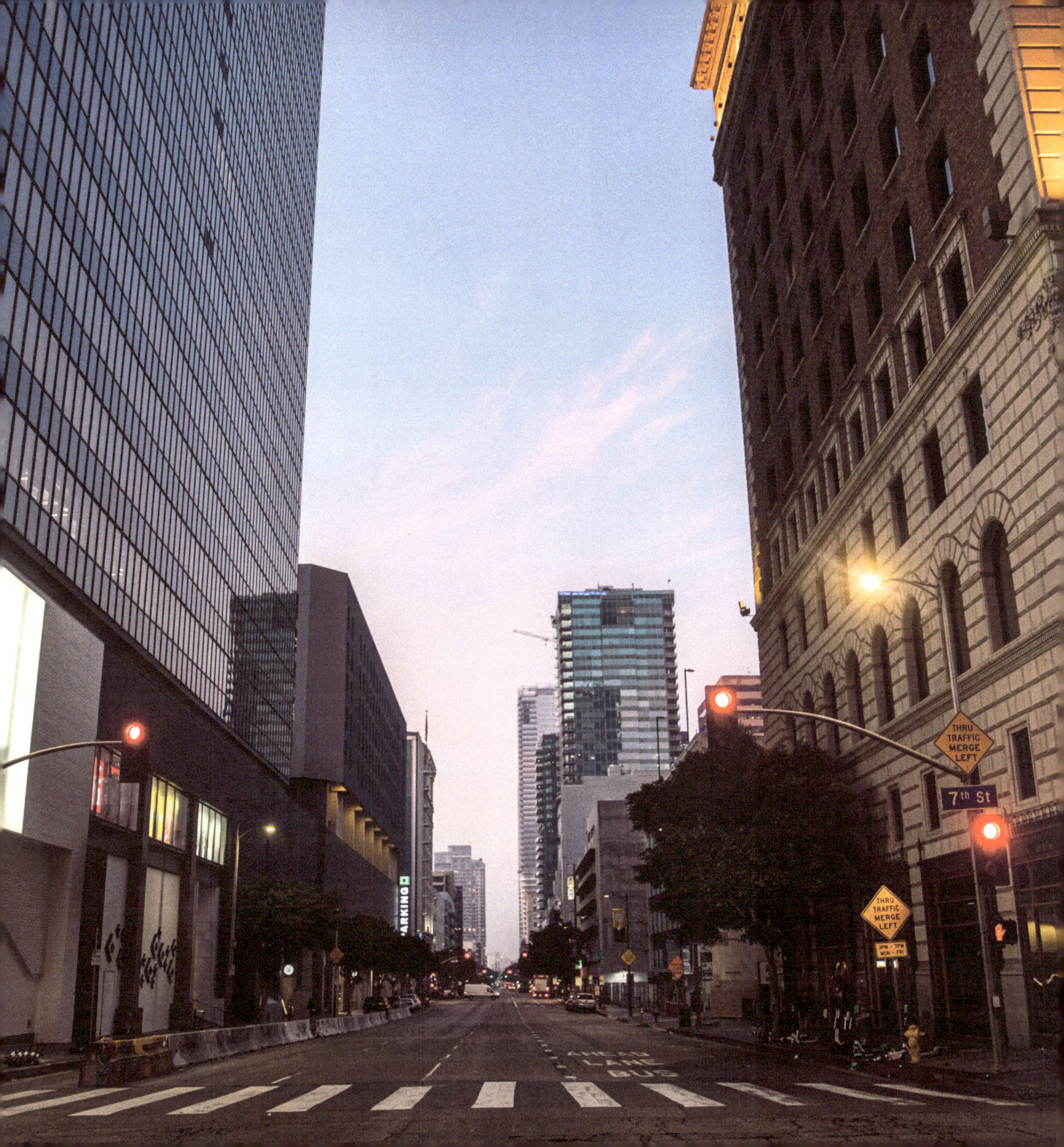
PARKING
THRU TRAFFIC MERGE LEFT
7th St
THRU TRAFFIC MERGE LEFT
3PM - 7PM MON - FRI
LANE
BUS

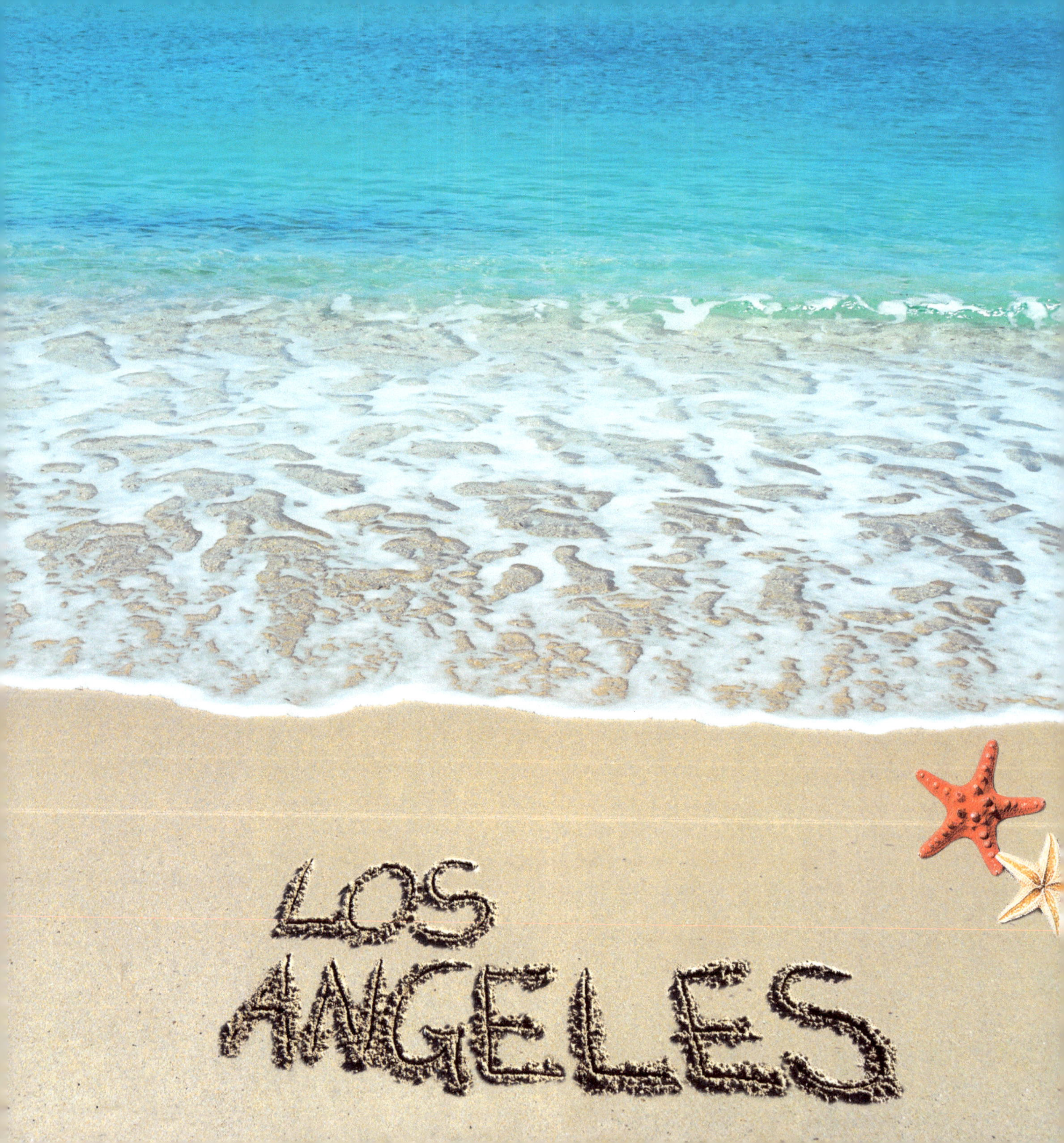

LOS
ANGELES